Sick & Tired Series

Help for the Sick & Tired

Advice, Encouragement, and Humor

From Those Who Understand

KIMBERLY RAE

Praise for
Sick and Tired

This is a MUST READ for anyone that has a chronic illness or knows someone with a chronic illness. It is well written and truly insightful. —Rhonda

Who would have thought that a book about chronic health issues would put a smile on a reader's face? But that's exactly what author Kimberly Rae has managed to elicit from this reader in her sometimes humorous, always compassionate, "Sick & Tired".... This short read is set up to be a perfect study guide for a group. As a Registered Nurse, I highly recommend this wonderful read. —Elaine

I read this book and wept. I wept at the understanding, I wept at the agreement and I wept at the hope and humor. I will be able to hand this to my family and friends and have what I have wanted to tell them, and what I wanted them to understand, explained in a gentle, compassionate and amusing way. —JD

Not "preachy" but very good encouragement with some practical tips as well. So glad I read it! —Diane

There were so many things in the book that resonated with what I go through.... she gets it! —Tammy

Why Doesn't God Fix It?

The chapter on depression was excellent. —Shades of REaD Book Club

Great book...It will encourage many. —Bethany

I like the scripture references and the applications. —Sue

This is a book that should be in every church's library. It would also make a very good text for a special Sunday School class or small-group read, particularly for any members suffering from a "why me?" response to their health concerns. —Lee Ashford of Reader's Favorite

Help for the Sick & Tired

Copyright © December 2019 by Kimberly Rae
www.kimberlyrae.com
Cover design by Kimberly Thigpen
All rights reserved.
For more information on this book, the author,
or permissions visit www.kimberlyrae.com

Library of Congress Cataloging-in-Publication Data
Rae, Kimberly.
Help for the Sick & Tired/ Kimberly Rae
Sick & Tired Series Book Four, Second Edition

Printed in the United States of America
ISBN: 9781707029143

Sick & Tired Series

<u>SICK & TIRED</u>
But You Don't Look Sick!
It's Not Fair—Giving Yourself Permission to Grieve
Losing Your Identity to Sickness
How to Explain Your Illness so People Don't Think You're Faking It

<u>YOU'RE SICK, THEY'RE NOT</u>
Chronic Illness Changes Relationships
Why Did God Do This to My Family?
Illness and Your Love Language
Chronic Illness and Your Personality Type

<u>WHY DOESN'T GOD FIX IT?</u>
Bribing God
The What Ifs and If Onlys
Illness and Depression
God I'll Trust You If…

<u>LAUGHTER FOR THE SICK & TIRED</u>
Funny Stories and Jokes, Just for Fun

<u>HELP FOR THE SICK & TIRED</u>
Choosing the Right Doctor
All the Advice you Never Wanted
To Church or not to Church
I Believe You

Available in paperback and e-book.

DEDICATION

To YOU

Table of Contents:

Strengthen the weak hands,
And make firm the feeble knees.
Say to those who
are fearful-hearted,
"Be strong, do not fear!"
Isaiah 35:3-4

INTRODUCTION

My biggest fear about becoming a zombie
is all the walking that I'd have to do.
Anonymous

I heard once about a study on pain endurance where test subjects had to stand in icy water while analysts calculated how long they could endure under different circumstances. In one scenario, the sufferer was able to endure twice as long as they normally would. This feat wasn't due to a pill or a program. It was if someone else was there encouraging them to keep going.

Imagine it with me. A person in pain, uncomfortable, sick and tired of sticking it out. She wants to quit, is about ready to give up, but then a friend or group of friends comes into the room.

They surround her.

"You can do this!" they call out.

"Hang on," one says. "One more minute. Keep going."

"Don't give up!"

That support is what this book is meant to be. No magic solution, just a group of us who know how it feels, offering what we can to help you endure and overcome. We'll give tips and commiserate a bit.

Most of all, we're cheering you on.

You can do this.
Hang on.
Don't give up!

That I may be encouraged together
with you by the mutual faith
both of you and me.
Romans 1:12

I want to be like a caterpillar.
Eat a lot, sleep for a while,
and then wake up beautiful.

Anonymous[i]

Bad

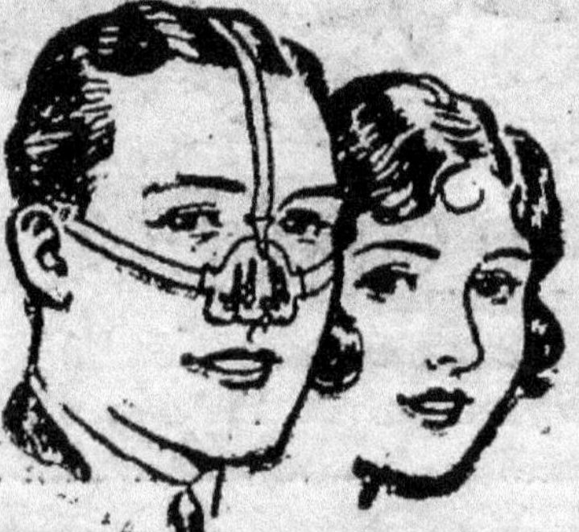

And after your nose is "permanently" fixed,
you can order the Lip Shaper too!

Worse

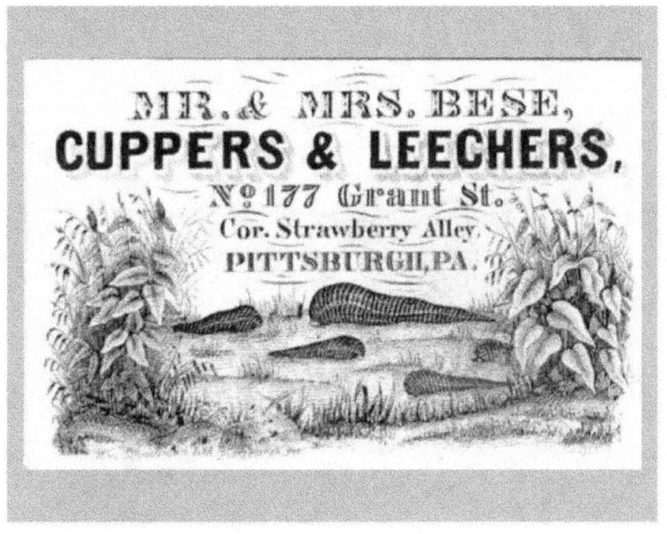

The latest medical treatment isn't always
the greatest medical treatment!

Heaviness in the heart of man
maketh it stoop:
but a good word maketh it glad.
Prov 12:25 KJV

CHAPTER ONE

I BELIEVE YOU

Be kind to people, and if that's too much
to ask for then just be weird to people.
It's the least you can do.
Anonymous[ii]

You know the look. Arched eyebrow. Pulled in chin. Grimacing smile. They don't believe you. It's possible the person is having a sudden attack of gout, but more likely he or she is listening to your symptoms and thinking, "Well, if you'd only…

clean up your diet
exercise
take this supplement
go organic
use essentials oils
have more faith
…you'd be fine."

Such moments, as much as we might not want them to, bring out our claws. Or maybe they open years of old wounds, unseen, throbbing, worse even than the hurt in our bodies. Anger and bitterness are the natural reactions. Or we want to spit out a little sarcasm, some cutting remark that lets them and everyone around them know how much their useless, self-propelled, you-don't-know-me-from-Eve's cousin advice is appreciated.

Gout or doubt, it won't do any good blowing up at people, or emotionally crumpling in a heap at their feet. Neither reaction is worth the personal cost.

Here's why:

Each of us is the epicenter of our universe. We can't help it. Even if we try, we cannot look at the world through someone else's eyes (unless we received them from a donor). We might walk a mile in their moccasins, but those shoes are never going to fit quite right, and we're still walking in them wherever *we* choose to go.

I will never fully understand you. You will never fully understand me, which is okay since a lot of times I don't understand myself! I could learn about you for the next ten years and still not be able to view life from your personal perspective.

When you mention your illness, that term or set of symptoms are never received in a vacuum, exclusive to the person listening. That person hears the words but they go into the filter of their own knowledge, experiences, assumptions and conclusions. Their response comes from their epicenter back to yours, for you to react out of your own knowledge, experiences, assumptions and conclusions.

What this means in plain English is that people think of themselves even when trying to think of others. You do it too. It's unavoidable—the brain inside your head is the only one you've got to work with.

For example, if you tell a group about your heart racing, the heart attack survivor, panic attack sufferer and cancer patient are all going to think of different possible causes and probably give different advice on what you should do.

Those who've never had a racing heart might be tempted to think you're being melodramatic, trying to get attention, or somehow creating the problem yourself by your bad eating habits or whatever.

It's certainly easier to decide a person is faking it than to recognize that each human is a magnificently complex creation of endless microscopic wonders, all combined to make them totally and irrevocably unique.

I think diagnosis labels have messed that up. Originally intended to help by defining a collection of problems that fit a certain pattern, the diagnosis now has become the boxed standard, forcing the sick person to fit the standard rather than the standard serving the person.

While unfortunate, this phenomenon isn't surprising. We humans love leaning on our own understanding, and though we are vastly ignorant of so much of our universe, from the colossal galaxies to the tiniest cells, we still have trouble admitting that something outside the box can be fully valid.

Hence the responses we sometimes get when X symptoms don't belong with Y symptoms, because they negate diseases A, B, and C. The tests and the book and the studies are to be trusted; therefore, since there cannot be a dearth in the results, there must be something wrong with us.

Bingo. That's what we've been saying all along. There's something wrong with us!

Nowhere in these pages will you read that…

- **Maybe you're faking it to get attention.** If we're going to fake something, why not pick something fun, like being a glowing unicorn that can fly backwards?

- **If you'd just _________________, you'd be fine.**

- **Thinking positively will fix everything.** Produce your own pixie dust and life will become a musical, in technicolor.

I want you to imagine telling me what you're going through, all of it, even the stuff you've stopped saying anymore to avoid that arched look. Here's space to write it if you want:

Now, picture me looking right at you from the pages of this chapter, and hear what I have to say:

I believe you.

You don't have to prove you're not lying by some graph or blood number or big long word that makes you officially sick.

I believe you.

You might be one number short of the line that makes professionals see your symptoms as valid, just one little number from getting the medicine you need.

I believe you.

You may be giving everything you've got and it still isn't seen as enough by those who should be most supportive and understanding.

I can't replace any of the above, but know that there are plenty of us who know the feeling of being more unique than we'd like to be, of baffling doctors and confusing friends and wishing we didn't need to prove ourselves so much and to so many.

You are completely unique, but you are not alone. You'll find people whose symptoms are as strange and off the grid as yours. If you don't believe me, keep reading.

Maybe we are sent to each other because we understand, not the condition necessarily, but the need. We can give the beautiful gift of believing each other. No eyebrows shooting toward the roof. No grimacing.

Some days, that really matters. Really helps.

I hope today is one of those days.

As one whom his mother comforts,
so I will comfort you.
God, Isaiah 66:13

Practical Page:

The "spoon theory" is my favorite way to show others life with chronic illness, particularly our need to make careful choices about how we spend our limited energy throughout the day.

The spoon metaphor for chronic illness was created by Christine Miserandino[iii] one day when a friend asked her what it was like living with lupus. They were sitting in a café, and Christine, trying to think of a way to explain such a complicated, varying situation, collected spoons from the nearby tables and had her friend hold them. She then had her friend describe actions throughout a normal day, taking away one of her spoons each time she used up energy for a task. The friend quickly ran out of spoons long before the day's typical activities could be completed.

Seeing this visual of Christine's struggle each day brought tears to the friend's eyes. I doubt she ever forgot that moment, and because it explains a large concept so clearly and succinctly in a way healthy people can understand, the spoon theory had become hugely popular among the chronic illness community, which is why you may encounter people referring to themselves as "spoonies" or mentioning how they ran out of spoons that day.

Legend says that
when you can't sleep,
it's because you're awake
in someone's dream.
So if everyone could stop
dreaming about me,
that would be great.

Anonymous[iv]

Bad

A Practical Invention That Develops Hair Growth

We have always maintained that if there were something that would really induce the hair to grow, its virtue should first be satisfactorily proved in each individual case before any money is paid to the manufacturer.

We have demonstrated beyond all question that in cases where the life-principle is not destroyed a reasonable use of our invention, THE EVANS VACUUM CAP, will develop a natural and permanent growth of hair, and we show our confidence by supplying this apparatus on a **sixty days' trial**, and wholly at our risk.

We would not have you infer from this that a complete restoration of the hair can be obtained within sixty days, but our experience shows that ample benefits usually accrue within this time to fully satisfy one as to the efficiency and practicability of this method.

It is simply an artificial means of obtaining a free and active circulation in the scalp, without rubbing or irritation, and there are no drugs or lotions employed.

The Cap is used three or four minutes each day, and it only requires about ten days to get the scalp loose and pliable, which condition is absolutely essential to the life and growth of the hair. The hair cannot thrive in a tight and congested scalp.

The effects produced by the vacuum are pleasant and exhilarating. It gives the scalp a healthy glow and produces a delightful tingling sensation, which denotes the presence of new life in the scalp, and which cannot be obtained by any other means. Channels which have been practically dormant for years are opened, and all follicle life is stimulated and revived to activity, and by supplying the hair roots with nutrition each day, in this way the weak, colorless hair is in time developed to its natural size and strength.

OUR GUARANTEE:

We will send you an EVANS VACUUM CAP by prepaid express, and will allow you sixty days to prove its virtue. As evidence of your good faith we simply ask that you deposit the price of the Cap with the Jefferson Bank, St. Louis, where it will remain during the trial period, pending the results of your experiment. This deposit is made subject to your own order, and, therefore, should you not be satisfied with the benefits derived you can of course instruct the Bank to return your money, which they will do promptly, and without question or comment.

Let us send you our book which describes and illustrates this appliance. Even if you are not in need of it, we know you will be interested in the invention, and what it has accomplished. The book is sent free on request.

THE EVANS VACUUM CAP CO., 505 Fullerton Building, St. Louis, U. S. A.

"We have demonstrated beyond all question that in cases where the life-principle is not destroyed…"

Nicely worded, so if it doesn't work,
it's your life-principle's fault.

Worse

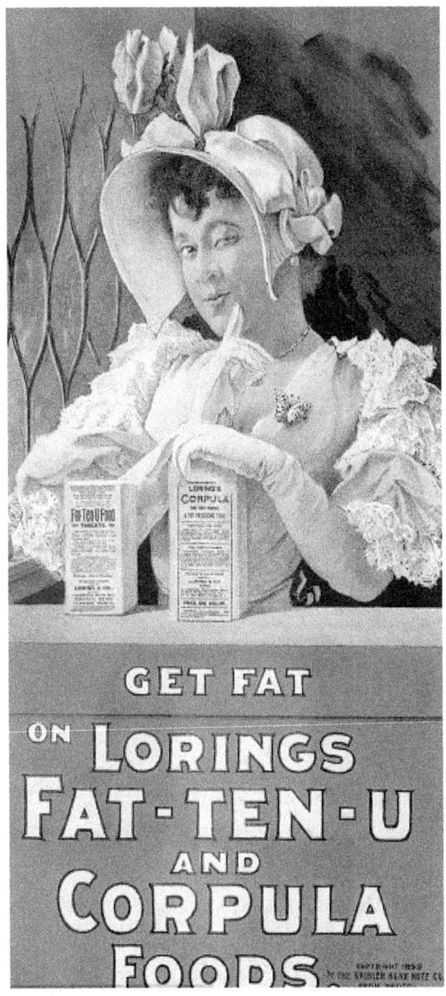

Haven't seen an ad on how to
make me fat in awhile!

Introducing…

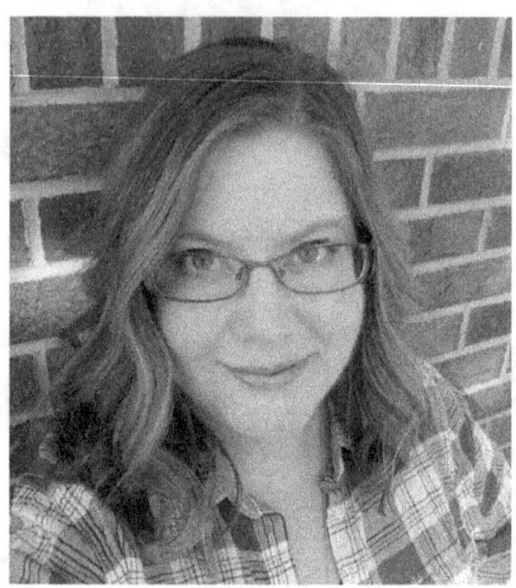

JD, like many of us, has a whole list of conditions, along with symptoms that have yet to belong to a label.

What diagnoses do you have so far?
I was diagnosed with hyper-coagulation syndrome pretty quickly. A blood clot from groin to ankle will do that. My other joint pain, migraines, dizziness, and fatigue they haven't bothered to diagnose.

How many doctors have you seen?
Wow...just GP's? Or just specialists? Or alternative? Probably fifteen GP's in the last eighteen years. I eventually stopped going when they demonstrated an utter lack of care in figuring out what's wrong with me. Specialists, I've probably seen ten or

more. Alternative healers, depends on your definition. I will say, conservatively, six. This doesn't even come close to counting lab techs who I have seen way more often than all the doctors combined.

But she doesn't look sick, does she?

*For You have considered
my trouble;
You have known my soul
in adversities....*
Psalm 31:7b

CHAPTER TWO

DO YOU LOOK SICK?

You just have to accept that some days
you are the pigeon,
and some days you are the statue.
Dr. Roger C Andersen[v]

"Oh, man, you look sick."

This, as we know, is a rude thing to say.

The opposite of rude is nice, so a reasonable assumption would be that to be nice, one should say the opposite, i.e. "You *don't* look sick."

The scenario plays out in real life.

Say Betty spends most of her energy getting ready for a party. By the time she gets there, she is depleted, but after years of practice is good at faking it.

Jean comes over to talk. After the initial small talk, they stand awkwardly, each in their own thoughts.

Betty is thinking:

I should have worn my practical shoes.

I wish I'd brought extra pain pills.

Is there a quiet place I could sit for a minute and recharge?

I want to congratulate Jean on her new job, but don't want her to feel sorry for me because I had to quit mine, or think I'm bringing it up out of envy.

I really should have worn my practical shoes.

Jean is busy with her own thoughts:

Wow, Betty looks so good. She must be doing a lot better than I'd heard. She's even wearing heels.

Should I ask her to help with my move next weekend? I don't want her to feel left out.

Then again, she never comes to anything I invite her to, so maybe I should skip it.

If she's doing so much better, why didn't she come to the church fellowship last Friday?

I wish I could ask her how she's really doing, but I feel stupid for not remembering the names of all the things she has. Does that make me a bad person?

I need to say something nice.

"So, Betty, how are you feeling lately?"

Betty would give her left toe to take off her shoes right now. "Oh, not too bad. You know."

No, Jean doesn't. She shrugs and half-smiles. "Well, you look great."

Betty drops eye contact, sure another person is telling her she's faking it. "Thanks."

Jean is grasping for something to say, but Betty seems to have shut down. "So I'm having a moving party next week. Want to come?"

Betty withdraws further. Why do people think she can lift heavy boxes? Doesn't anybody know her? Or care? "Oh, well, I'm busy then, but thanks."

Jean sighs. She should have known better than to ask. "Well, I see Bob over there. Better go say hi."

Betty slips out the back door and leaves the party early. Jean sighs and tells Bob, "I just don't think Betty likes being around people. Or at least not around me."

⌃

Can we fix this scenario? Yes, I think we can.

I propose an idea, not one I thought of myself, more like one that forced itself on me.

These days, I have to wear a breathing mask often, thanks to my brain surgery giving me a superhuman sense of smell, and thus making my asthma triggers that much more eager to ignite. Places with carpet, paper, or wood, like libraries or churches or homes, are difficult for me, as are people with any kind of scent on them. This is a complicated maze to maneuver in and around, especially because the problems are airborne and though some are obvious, like a person smoking, many are invisible until it's too late, like menthol rubs or fabric softener.

Wearing a mask can be cool for the star in a Marvel comic, or, say, Darth Vader. My mask looks like it belongs to Vader's albino twin. I have a cute one with flowers on it that's less intimidating, but also less effective, so the more sensitive my lungs get, the more scary the mask gets. I'm about on Phantom of the Opera level now, especially when I have to add gloves to actually touch the paper too.

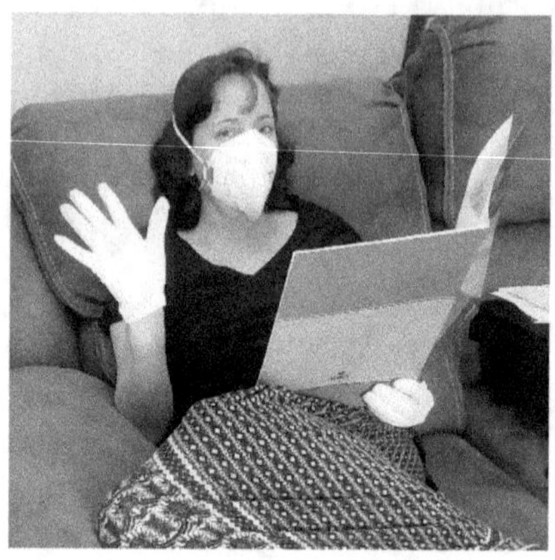

I can remember the first time I wore a mask in public. It was to a Chick-Fil-A with relatives over a holiday, and I was humiliated and embarrassed for myself and for them. In the years since then, I've gotten used to needing it at times, but this past year it has been prevalent. If I'm not going to Walmart or fast-food restaurants, or sitting inside my van, I can expect to need to wear it. I'm probably getting to be one of the most recognizable women in my small town, and not for my southern charm.

My masked adventures have been a kinetic lesson, however, in effective indirect communication. Wearing a mask tells people "I am sick." I think it also tells people one of two things:

1.   "I am contagious and might have the plague. Avoid me or pay the price."

2.   "I am fragile and should be treated gently."

One day at the Post Office, I tried to tell the lady behind the counter what I needed, but she was having trouble understanding through my mask, so I pulled it down to speak more clearly. I hadn't thought about how that might look until I saw the woman's eyes widen and her head went back ever so slightly. I could almost see the internal battle waging in her mind between wanting to back faaaar away from this potentially harmful creature, but not wanting to be obvious about it. I almost milked that moment of power, but had pity and told her I wasn't contagious; it was only an asthma flair.

At least I think I did. Maybe I didn't and she ran right out and got a flu shot.

Back to if we have to look sick. This starts out as a major negative. It draws attention to the fact that we are sub-normal, and feels like we're begging for pity, things we work hard to avoid.

But when we succeed in faking it, we suffer the consequences, like people assuming we can go to this event because we showed up at that one, or they see us looking fine today so assume we must be feeling fine also.

The mask cured that for me. It is a big sign to people, an instant way of saying, "I have health struggles. Take that into consideration when interacting with me, okay?"

It has also provided surprising benefits, like:

1. **People don't stare.** Little kids do, but I'm fine with that. Other people glance, then quickly look away so they aren't rude. My mask creates my own

little introvert bubble to walk around in. Some days that's a blessing.

2.   **People don't expect as much.** Who's going to ask a girl who looks fragile to take over the nursery schedule or organize the Christmas play? It offers an immediate set of boundaries I don't have to verbalize.

3.   **It provides extra personal space at yard sales and stores.** People don't tend to hover over sickies who wear masks. This I enjoy immensely.

4.   **I don't have to wear makeup.** I miss getting to pretend I'm normal sometimes, but it's a plus to get to look as tired as I want because no one can see most of my face anyway.

5.   **It's a good diet tool.** One of my masks got a brown dot in the middle because I was cooking and wanted to taste the teriyaki sauce!

6.   **People remember my limitations more.** "Oh yeah, there's that girl with the breathing problem. Better not go near her if you're wearing that nice-smelling deodorant. If you stink, though, you're okay."

7.   **It reminds me I'm sick.** My default is to want to fake it, but it's hard to fake being normal when you've got a white blanket strapped to your face.

Application? Get yourself a mask for the bad days, or a cane, or a sling or brace or anything that shows without you having to explain to everyone, and then explain again when they forget, and then feel badly that they feel badly, etc. If you don't have any good reason for a cane or walker or whatever, carry around a prescription bottle with a bottle of water, one in each hand so you have to shift things around every time you shake hands with someone. Okay, that one might be over the top, but I'm serious about getting something that visibly shows people you have limitations.

I know it's hard. Feels like we're making a production of our illness, but it actually keeps us from having to make a production of it. We don't have to talk about it if it's right there to see. And if we have something obvious, it's a conversation topic. It gives people a way to ask about how we're doing without feeling as awkward.

Let's try it with Betty and Jean.

Betty comes to the party with a brace around her ankle and her wrist.

Jean comes to talk. "Oh my goodness. What happened?"

"Nothing." Betty smiles and shrugs. "My joints flare up when a storm comes through. The braces help with the pain and keep me from pulling ligaments." Another smile and a point. "But look, I still got into my favorite pair of heels!"

Jean laughs with her. "You're amazing. I love your perspective. So do you always have to wear a brace when there's a storm?"

Betty invites Jean to sit with her. "Do you really want to know? I don't want people to think I'm always talking about it."

"Oh no, I'm really curious, I just didn't want to be nosey."

Both Betty and Jean leave the party with the promise to get together again soon, some sunny day when Betty's feeling good. Betty feels great that she doesn't have a commitment she'll probably have to break, because getting together will be spontaneous, sometime when she's in a good spot, and Jean is happy because she's learning how to be Betty's friend within her limitations.

It doesn't always work so smoothly, but the potential is there. Having a visual "sick" sign can give you and others a reference point, a focus, a springboard for conversation. Do you see how it could help? Wouldn't you like it if some of your friends with chronic illness had something visible that reminded you of their limitations? We don't need to walk around in a plastic bubble or anything, but something small, something that shows, could spark the start of big positive change.

Finally, all of you be of one mind, having compassion for one another…be tenderhearted, be courteous.
1 Peter 3:8

Practical Page:

Rent the wheelchair.
Wear the mask.
Use the cane.
Scrap the heels and pick comfy shoes.
Make the choices you can to make it easier, so you can focus more on people and less on pain.

I have an air couch "blob" that makes it possible for me to go to an outdoor event that has no squishy seating options. It looks silly, but works, and I think all the cool-looking people in their uncomfortable seats secretly envy me.

28

Laughing is like changing
a baby's diaper.
It doesn't solve any problems
permanently,
but it makes things more
acceptable for awhile.

Barbara Johnson[vi]

Bad

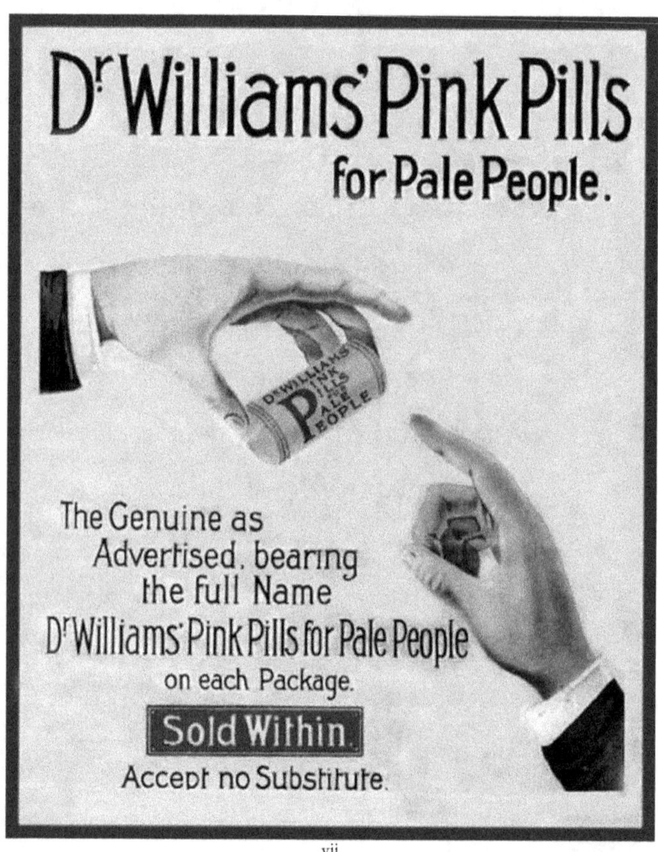

vii

Are these to make pale people pink?

Worse

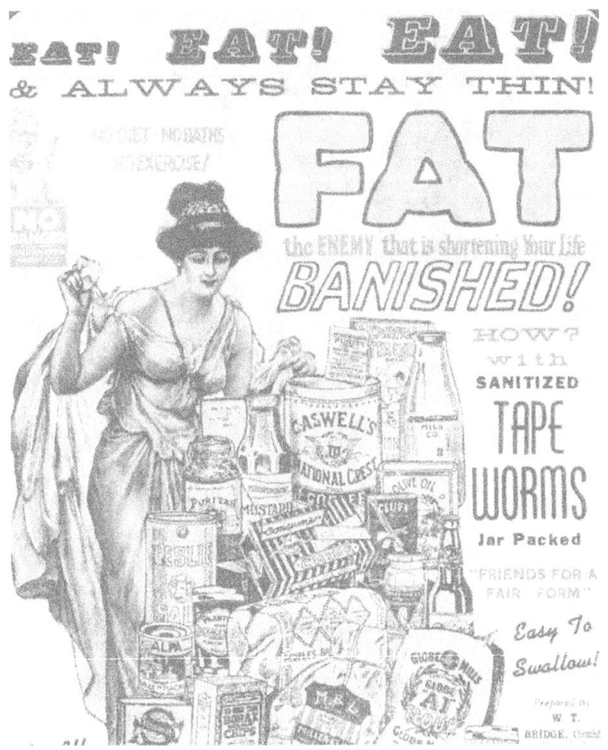

How do they make any tapeworm,
sanitized or not, easy to swallow?!
I guess these are for the people who took too much
of the Fat-En-U stuff from the last chapter.

Introducing…

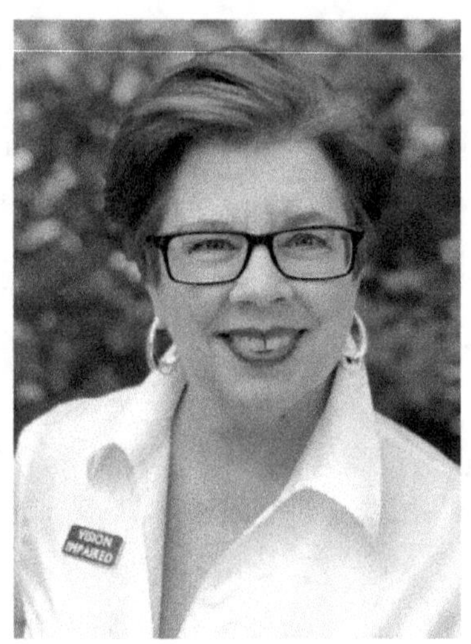

Patricia interviews Christian writers and speakers every weekday on her Facebook page, *Marketers On A Mission*. She looks perfectly healthy so I forget she's limited until I see the badge she wears that says: Vision Impaired.

It's simple, not ostentatious or asking for attention, and very effective.

Bravo, Patricia! Let's find out more.

What is something someone said that helped you?

I've always had poor eyesight. I'm legally blind in one eye and have Keratoconus in the other eye. Both continue to progress every year. I began wearing the badge in the late 90's, when flying to a Christian writers conference alone. I asked Christ for help to maneuver through the airport and conference crowds without being run over. He suggested this solution. (All His ideas are good.)

I purchase my badges from a local trophy shop. They're magnetized so they don't make a hole in my garments. I wear one anytime I'm out in public. They explain to people—without me saying a word—why I need extra help to read price tags in stores, why I ask questions when a sign with the answer is nearby, why I can't find what I'm searching for in the library, and so forth. It allows me to move about freely in environments that would otherwise be closed off to me, so it's been a major improvement in my life. I give Him the praise for it.

I have heard many such things;
Miserable comforters are you all!
Shall words of wind have an end?
Or what provokes you that you answer?

I also could speak as you do,
If your soul were in my soul's place.
I could heap up words against you,
And shake my head at you;

But I would strengthen you
with my mouth,
And the comfort of my lips
would relieve your grief.
Job 16:1-5

CHAPTER THREE

ALL THE ADVICE YOU NEVER WANTED

An apple a day keeps anyone anyway,
if you throw it hard enough.
Anonymous[viii]

Advice. How do you feel when you hear that word coming out of someone's mouth?

Dread is the word that comes to my mind. *Oh no, here it comes. Something I've probably tried three times already, or that has nothing to do with my actual condition. Keep smiling. Nod your head. Work up the energy to explain why this isn't going to become your instant next life priority. Should I tell them about my notebook bulging with all the things I've tried and terrible side effects they caused or money spent or hopes I've had dashed? Should I simply say thanks and move on, but then be aware they might ask next week if I've tried it yet?*

Can I just go home?

Likely you and I both have days when we're up for being an ambassador of information and don't mind receiving the well-intentioned suggestions from people who wish we were better and wish they knew a way to help us get there. Other days, like maybe today because you're reading this and I'm writing it, we're just so tired. Too tired of living it to explain it to one more, two more, six more people.

I feel a sense of regret regarding this. Connection through talk is how women build deep relationships. Maybe that's part of it, actually. Pardon me if I think on paper for a minute. If a close friend gives a suggestion, I appreciate that because I know they know what I have and care. The random ones feel kind of like strangers walking up and saying, "I want to be your new friend! Come for a jog with me and tell me all about yourself." I don't have the umph to jog with my closest friends, so it's extra draining to have to respond well and kindly and with energy to the randoms. Hmm, maybe defining what kind of advice-giver is facing us would make it easier to form a proper, or less-wearying, response.

I think best in visual metaphor, so let's look at advice givers within a totally different setting, like sports.

Types of People Who Offer Advice

Couch Potato Spectator: Doesn't know anything about the sport, they just like to hear themselves talk.

Response: Smile and move on, do not put stock into their opinions or suggestions.

Grapevine Spectator: Gets together with others, thinks it's fun to throw out ideas and theories and pass along things they've heard without bothering to check if they have any validity. They want to be heard and feel guilty if they don't share something that might end up being helpful.

Response: Don't explain or defend; it's not about your personal condition. They want to offer whatever possible ideas they've heard or read, so acknowledge you got the info, which releases them to chase the next idea. I like to say, "I'll look that up." Then I look it up, confirm it won't work, and move on with my life. Sometimes an idea ends up helping, so it's worth checking.

Fan: Knows a little-to-fair bit about the sport so sees themselves as knowledgeable, but doesn't play the sport themselves. They are the hobby researchers or sellers or even counselors. They know a lot and can be helpful, but in the end it's outside their experience.

Response: Same as above. Check on their suggestions if you want, but don't feel you have to explain why it did or didn't work.

Newest Fad or Fear: The kind that says, "Back in the day, a spoonful of ___________ was all we needed," or, "Michael Phelps does cupping so of course it would work for you." They're not thinking about the fact that "back in the day" remedies could contain anything from whiskey to heroin, and just because something worked for a celebrity, or a million people, doesn't mean it will work for you. Often these people are recommending things more on emotional response to the latest cool trend or even a fear tactic. ("Don't try that one! My cousin's sister's neighbor heard of someone who tried it and her face exploded!")

Response: I recommend distraction technique on this one. Jump to a story of another who-knows-who that tried such-and-such and had a reaction, or ask a question that lets them talk about it, or simply say, "How interesting," and change the subject.

Rookie: The ones who recently started on a new treatment and are convinced it is the cure-all for everyone on the planet. They feel a great energy from all the success stories and even their own initial positive response. Not to be a downer, but I've tried many a thing that helped for a time, but the benefits faded as the core problem overrode the initial systemic response.

Response: Don't squash their zeal, but don't jump in either. I recommend finding someone who has been on it for over a year and seeing how the results stand up to long-term usage. If it doesn't tend to last, I don't think it will help to try to explain it; wait and time will do the explaining for you.

Former Athlete: Has helpful tips and is good to learn from, but their insights come from their own experience.

Response: Unless you've hired them as a personal coach, listen to the advice as info but don't feel you have to follow it.

Coach: Aha! A good one is a former athlete who understands what it's like, is still active in the sport, keeps up with changes over time, and wants to help as part of a winning team. These are the mentors you want to find. They're rare, but valuable.

Response: Can we talk?

ಌ

It is only right to say here that I am not bashing advice giving, just a frustration over advice without relationship or knowledge. My life was probably saved by a personal message on Facebook once, and there have been a couple of other suggestions that have hugely helped my condition. To all the people who genuinely care and give ideas out of love and a desire to help, sincere thanks to them. To the others, they're probably not reading this anyway, so we can smile and move on.

He who is slow to wrath
has great understanding.
Prov 14:29

Practical Page:

Advice is like a drug. It has side effects for the person who has to swallow it, but doesn't hurt the person who gives it. If it's for a condition you have, it could be hugely helpful…or not. If it's for something you don't have, it can have terrible consequences if you try it. For the random person who shoves something at you, those are best flushed down the nearest toilet. Don't carry them around in a bag that gets heavier and heavier over time, eventually causing you a new condition!

According to hospital insurance codes,
there are 9 different ways
you can be injured by turtles.

Wall Street Journal

Bad

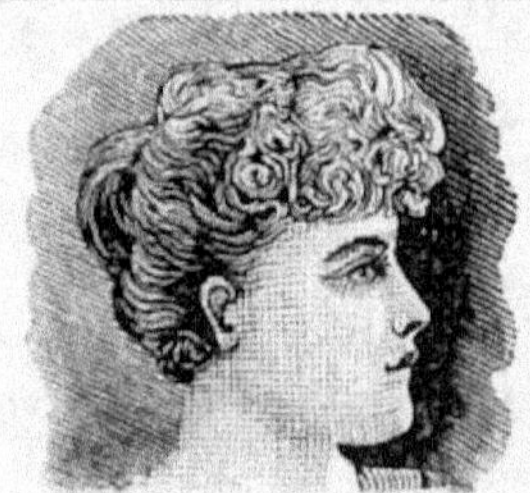

Dearie, I think your freckles and pimples
will become a minor problem
when your face starts disintegrating.

Worse

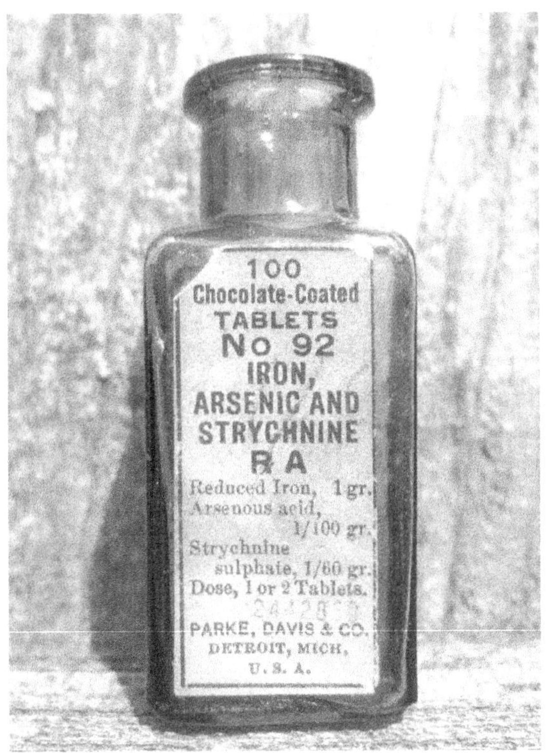

And a chocolate-coated option
in case you like your poison flavored.

Introducing…

Marie has had Multiple Sclerosis for almost 40 years. She wrote this prayer before an MS relapse and grueling pain for twenty-two days.

"Here I Am Again"
Father, here I am again.
I finally realize why I've been downcast
for the last few days.
I should recognize this familiar place.
For days now there has been a pattern
of sleep without rest;
of dragging fatigue;
of forcing myself to smile when I need to;
of searching for a comfortable way to sit;
of struggling to remember names;
of staring at the computer
without being able to write;
of feeling weepy and withdrawn
without apparent reason.

Here I am again.
The painful buzzing in my legs this morning
signaled yet another MS relapse.
I just checked my calendar.
I went into relapse at almost
the exact same week last year.

Somehow, figuring out the reason for my despondency
has lifted my spirits.
Now I have a familiar battle to fight,

and I know what weapons to use.
I cling to Your Word, my Lord.
"Why are you downcast, oh my soul?"
cried David in the Psalms.
Then He took refuge in praise.
So will I, my glorious Father!
You have said in Your Word
that You inhabit the praise of Your people.
I choose to praise You,
O glorious Lord!
You have a reason to set me
in a quiet place now.
It is here, in this time aside with You,
that You will teach me
and minister to my very soul.

So I welcome this relapse.
May it be a time of respite and renewal.
May I praise You with song
and with mediating on Your promises.
May every sting of pain be a reminder
of what Christ endured for me.
May every sleepless night be filled
with listening to You.
May my foggy mind be filled
instead with the clarity of Your glory.
May my exhausted body find refreshment
as I drink from Your Word.
May I come forth with fresh vision
and strength to do Your will.
So I will meet You in the arbor,
where You will prune this branch.
I love You, Lord.

For I, the Lord your God,
will hold your right hand,
Saying to you,
"Fear not, I will help you."
Isaiah 41:13

CHAPTER FOUR

LAURA'S STORY
In her words, by Laura Smith

Hope is the feeling you have
that the feeling you have isn't permanent.
Barbara Johnson [ix]

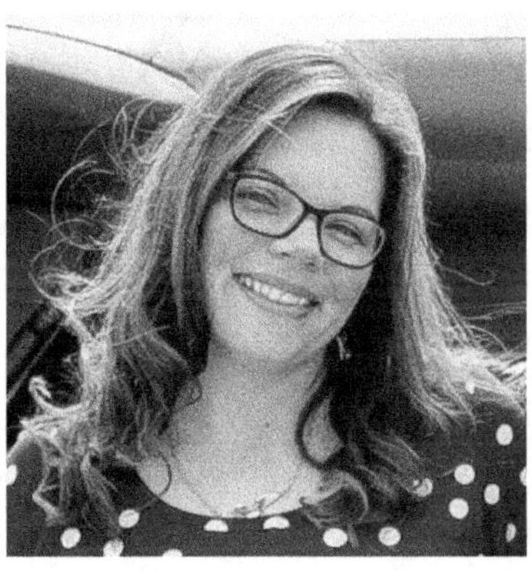

My health journey began long ago, though I didn't realize it. I can now trace my symptoms back to when I was a young child. It has been within the last several years that light has been shed onto the mysterious illnesses that hold my body captive most days. My official diagnoses are: Generalized Anxiety Disorder, Panic Disorder, Postural Orthostatic Tachycardia Syndrome (POTS), Fibromyalgia, Myalgic Encephalomyelitis (M.E.), Chronic Small Intestinal Bacterial Overgrowth (SIBO) from toxic mold build up and growth inside my body, Ehlers-Danlos (EDS) and Central Diabetes Insipidus (this is not related to Type 1 or 2 Diabetes). This has been a long, hard journey. When my symptoms began to be disabling a few years ago, I knew there was something much bigger going on than daily stress and fatigue.

I began by seeing my family physician who felt I was dramatizing my symptoms. As is the case with many military dependents, my primary care physician changed often, with no warning. Every time this happened, I would go in for a visit with the hopes of finally getting someone who would listen. Each time led to disappointment. Out of pity or more likely annoyance at my continual visits and pleas for help, someone would throw in a referral for an MRI, X-ray, or more bloodwork. And each would be mostly inconclusive, neutral or find small imbalances that nobody felt were big enough to address.

Once, I was explaining to a new doctor all my symptoms, my history, my diagnoses, and after 10 minutes or so, she handed me the clipboard and asked me to fill my own chart out! She said not only could she not keep up with what I was telling her, she didn't know what half of my diagnoses were!

Time progressed and I felt worse with each passing day. At an agonizingly slow pace, I did start to find some guidance. I was diagnosed with POTS after I passed out and fell off a table in a physician's office. I saw a rheumatologist who was able to identify Ehlers-Danlos, Fibromyalgia and M.E. A neurologist discovered the Central Diabetes Insipidus accidentally when he was digging into my POTS issues. Several more years down the road, a Functional Medicine

Practitioner questioned if it was my mast cells misbehaving wildly and began treatment. This ended up being the wrong road and did, for a time, cause me to become more sick than I have ever been; however, it did put me on the path to being honest with myself and others and come to terms with struggles with anxiety.

Can I take the briefest of moments here and tell you mental health is not something to be taken lightly? There is such a heavy stigma with talking about anxiety and depression and it really needs to stop. We shouldn't be made to feel guilty, embarrassed or less than because we struggle with these. We should be able to embrace what it is, acknowledge it and ask for the proper help, without hesitation. It took me far too long to understand this truth. I now know, how left unchecked, these issues can arise in very physical manifestations. To be completely vulnerable here, I will tell you that once I was told I must not actually be a Christian because Christians don't experience anxiety. God brought His truth to light for me and showed me 1 Peter 5:7 which says, "cast all your anxieties on him, because he cares for you." He wouldn't have made sure this would be in the Bible, if He didn't already know we would need to know this truth as the broken humans that we are.

I am, or I used to be, a go-getter, a "type-A," thrive on that to-do list type woman. I was busy, I was productive. I had big goals and dreams. Then it all came to a screeching halt. The migraines became constant. The pain set into my joints. Waves of nausea followed by uncontrollable vomiting were a new norm. The dizziness became more frequent as did the heart palpitations, inconsistent blood pressure, visual changes, and every other symptom that goes along with these illnesses. I wish I could tell you my faith has been big in this. I wish I could tell you I didn't falter once. I wish I could say that in my hardest moments I remembered an inspiring Scripture verse to help me through but that would be a lie. At best I have been mediocre. At moments, I have screamed out to God in complete and utter anger and cried myself to sleep on the bathroom floor. I have picked up my Bible and quickly put it back down again to replace it with anything else that might not expose truth and therefore expose my ugliness and sin. I have definitely tried to reason with Him many, many times, that He messed this one up. He was wrong about allowing what was happening in my body and where my life was headed.

I have been through all the stages of grief many times over the years and each cycle brings with it new growth. I have finally come to a place of acceptance, but it really is God's grace and mercy that has allowed me to be where I am today. I was wildly stubborn, and He had to break me to mold me. I wanted things that were not part of His plan for me. Do I think He created me with these health complications? No. But I do think He allowed them and continues to allow them to make me more Christ-like. And isn't that the point? To know Him and make Him known? And how can we make Him known when we don't know Him outside our small idea of who He is and how He fits into our premediated idea of how our lives are going to be?

I fought long and hard to find peace with my new limitations. But I am grateful to share with you I am much closer to achieving it than I have ever been! I've even found joy and humor in this constantly changing journey. You see, I wanted to be busy and productive and constantly achieve new goals. I was doing that, but at a cost. I was missing a lot of the little things that were right in front of me. Where I thought I wanted busy and fast, He gave me mindful and slow. He brought the small things into a clear, sharp focus where I once zipped right past without the slightest idea something was there. I wanted to be seen. To be recognized. I thought that's where I was headed and maybe I was, but to whose glory? Mine. Where I wanted to be seen and heard for my own selfish reasons, He gave me a quiet time-out to see the error in my heart. He gave me a time of solitude and allowed many of my "friends" to walk away from me because of my limitations so I could find my worth and recognition in Him and Him alone.

I yearned to accomplish something great in my life. I thought that looked like paper certificates, acceptance speeches, medals, and trophies. I thought it looked like climbing my way to the top with ruthless zeal. I was so, so wrong. Though every lesson along the way has had purpose and added tremendous value to my life, this has been the most valuable yet: My greatest accomplishment in life will never be something I do on my own. It is simple and it is profound, and it is eternal. It is to love the Lord my God with all my heart, with all my soul, with all my strength, and with all my mind, and my neighbor as myself (see Luke 10:27). To love Him this way is to trust Him. To ask Him for guidance when things are hard. To let Him be my strength not only when I am weak, but always. To know with absolute certainty anything that comes my way is already handled and I have nothing to fear. To love Him like this means I love myself too. That I love myself the way He loves me. Without condition. Loving myself even when my body fails, when my mind is cloudy and confused, when I eat applesauce and chicken broth for days on end because I can't digest or tolerate anything else. To love Him like this means that the same love overflows from me into those around me. Into my wonderful husband, into my precious children, into the few family and friends that are in my life. It flows into interactions with neighbors, with those at church, with strangers. It flows through the very words you are reading, right into you. To love Him this way means spreading His love by simply loving. He has used these painful and depleting illnesses to teach me to love better. To love with a genuine heart.

I know many with illnesses struggle with fear. Loving so wholly helps to conquer fear. For me it was fear of the unknown. Fear of not knowing if there will be new symptoms or worsening symptoms or if these illnesses will lead to new ones. Fear of becoming completely disabled or losing more mobility. Fear of ruining my children's childhood because I'm not the mother I imagined I would be. Fear of over-burdening my husband with my constant restrictions and needs. Fear of not recovering from one of my body's attempts to destroy itself and leaving this place before I get a chance to see my husband grow old and my children settle into adulthood. Love conquers fear and let me tell you, He loves you and He loves me more than we will ever understand. He loves us so much that if He needs to allow our world to be turned upside down to help us find our way to Him more truly, He will, but He doesn't leave us to do it on our own. He is with us always. In the doctor's office when the news isn't what we had hoped, when the pain runs rampant through our body, when our tears flow heavy and leave us exhausted. He is there when there is momentary but blessed relief, when a cure is found, when a smile is shared in the treatment center, when a life is touched by our raw vulnerability in sharing our story and even when one life ends here and begins in His eternal kingdom.

I pray sharing this tiny piece of my journey brings you hope. That it brings you encouragement and fills your heart with beautiful and overwhelming love.

There is no fear in love;
but perfect love casts out fear,
because fear involves torment.
1 John 4:18

Practical Page:

<u>Laura's Tip:</u>
I keep a journal of prayers and gratitude. On my really hard days, it helps me to focus my attention on others by praying for their needs and when I am done with that, I write the things I am grateful for one by one. Sometimes I journal it through tears, sometimes between waves of nausea and other times with one eye open, lying sideways on the floor because my migraines can be super intense. Doing this helps me keep my mind in a good place, helps me still be able to love others by praying for them when I often can't leave my home, and helps me still find joy and blessing in hard moments and days.

<u>Advice she's heard and wants to pass along to you:</u>
Just take each day one moment at a time and extend grace to yourself as you go. You aren't who you once were and you can't hold yourself to the same expectations as you once did.

Overheard in Sunnyside Clinic, Fratton,
as a receptionist spoke to an
obviously hard-of-hearing client,
"No, Mrs. Jones,
not the HEARSE,
I'm sending the NURSE." ˣ

Bad

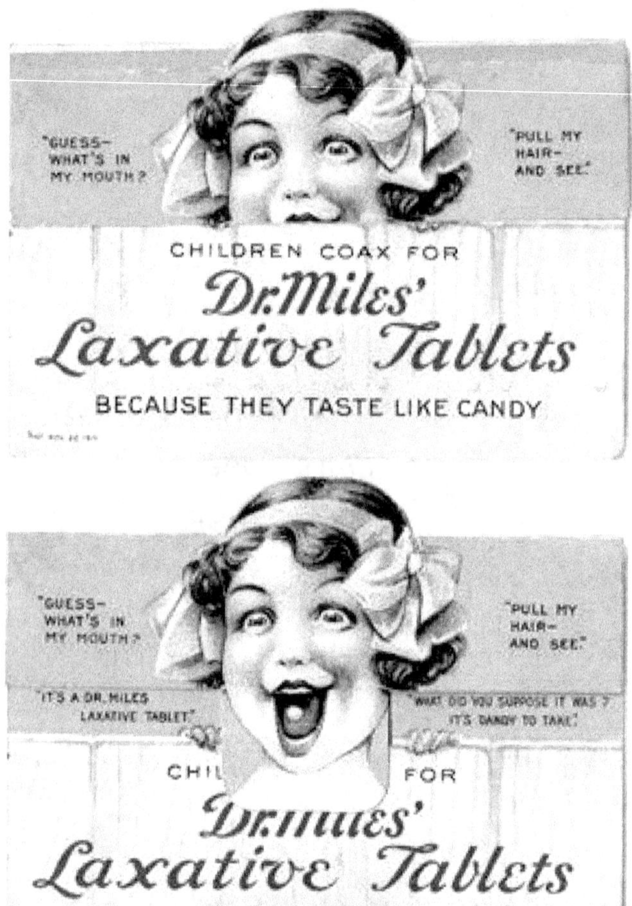

Why exactly do we want kids
eating laxatives like candy?

Worse

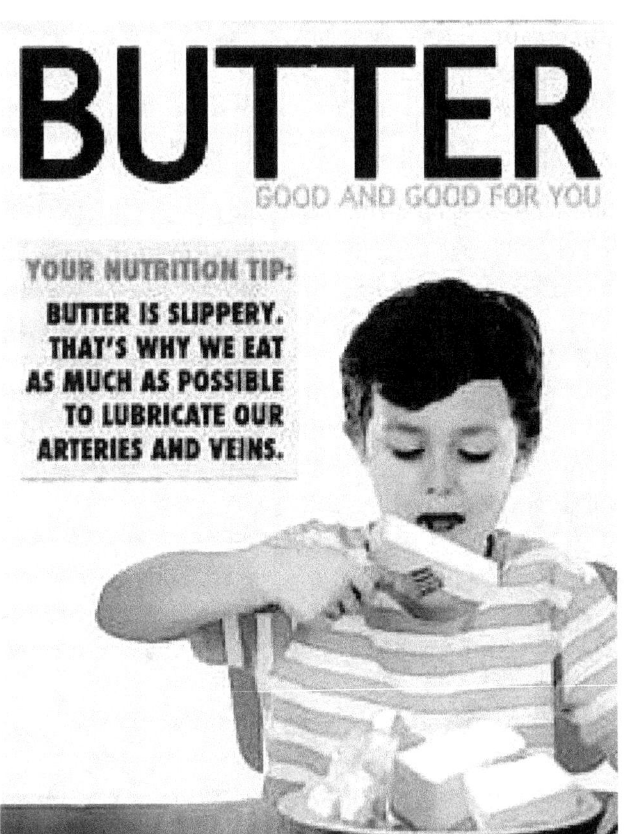

This explains so much.

Introducing…

Phyllis says of her husband, "To so many, my husband Bill didn't look sick. ('I saw Bill today and he looked so good,' or, 'I talked to Bill today and he sounded so good.') My answer may be, 'Oh, yes, he is good at faking it,' or just, 'Yes, he does.'"

Bill has Paget's bone disease, diabetes, and D.I.S.H. (arthritic disease - causes fusion of cervical discs). He gets infections, cellulitis and diabetic ulcers. He also experiences bouts of dementia or sundowners. Bill "had two back surgeries and no relief of pain since then. The pain caused him to withdraw from church and our social life. His counselor said, 'Bill, because of your constant pain, you have no reserve energy to deal with people.'"

<u>Who do they like to get advice from?</u>
Only those who have been there/done that, not those who say I hurt my back once and I understand.

<u>Does it help talking with others with the same issues?</u>
Bill hasn't found much comfort from others. But he has found great comfort in God and His Word. He has a deeper experience in the Lord than when his trial began 35 years ago.

<u>How do they bear it?</u>

We sometimes wonder if this experience is just what kept us close to the Lord and in the right way. We will never know but we have grateful hearts.

He shall not be afraid
of evil tidings:
His heart is fixed,
trusting in the Lord.
Psalm 112:7 KJV

CHAPTER FIVE

CRISIS, HOSPITALIZATION, AND RECOVERY

How is a hospital gown like insurance?
You're never as covered as you think you are. [xi]

If I asked you to tell me about a health crisis, what would come to mind? A recent scare? New, unexplained symptoms? A trip to the ER or hospital stay? Surgery? Being denied surgery?

Multiple scenarios could apply, but each of us has our own line that, when crossed, constitutes a crisis. Your line may not be in the same place as someone else's, which can cause hurt and frustration if that someone else happens to be a family member or doctor in charge of your care.

I'll skip sharing my stories as I'm sure you have your own. Yours might be of crossing your line and hitting a crisis, but others around you did not feel it valid enough for action. Or you might be on the opposite end, where others are pushing you toward a treatment or doctor visit you don't feel is necessary yet. Either way, the last time to deal with different approaches to crisis is in the middle of one.

We cannot always prevent crisis' from occurring, but we can prepare an action plan for them. Having a pre-determined plan is like creating a last will and testament. It helps make sure what is most important to you is prioritized.

Having an agreed-on plan with a doctor or caregiver or family members alleviates the need to:

- Convince them you're in crisis when it happens.
- Create a plan in the middle of the crisis, when you will not be as emotionally or mentally resourced.
- Deal with differing opinions at a time when relationship conflict should *not* be the priority.

Ideas for creating a crisis plan:

1.   **Define Crisis.** I was able to get clear, exact numbers from a doctor on what point to use my inhaler for asthma, what point to do additional self-treatment, and what point to go to the ER. That took away that horrible guessing game during an attack, when my body is panicking and my reasoning skills have taken a backseat.

For family members or caregivers, sitting down to a scheduled meeting during a non-crisis time and discussing each person's definition of what constitutes a crisis can help in understanding people's response or lack of response when you cross your crisis line. Agreeing on a crisis line can take away a great deal of stress and put everyone on the same starting line.

2.   **Define it for each of your conditions.**

Example:

Blood sugar below ___________ or above ___________.

Symptoms of _______________________ or visual cues of
_______________________.

3.   **Define exactly what you want people to do in response to the crisis.** Use if-then statements.
Example:
If I say I need to go to the ER for an asthma attack, trust me and take me. Please don't ask me a bunch of questions.
If my face starts swelling and I seem to be choking, give me a shot from my EpiPen, then take me to the ER.

4.   **Include helpful instructions.**
Example:
One EpiPen is in my black purse, another is in the glove compartment of my van. Instructions for giving shot are on the outside of the pen.

Keep these pages accessible, and if you find yourself crossing the line, you can get the appropriate page out, hand it over, and point. You could even make a version for your phone or computer that you could send via text or email when you need help from someone specific, or have it on your phone to show an ER doctor when you get there.

Your plan may morph over time, as you realize that, depending on the crisis, your desires may flip to the exact opposite of what you expected they would be, and that's okay. This is to get you started.

Beyond the Crisis
to Hospitalization and Recovery

In a crisis, your help typically comes from whoever is present with you when it happens. If the crisis turns into something bigger and longer, like surgery or a hospital stay, hopefully family, friends, neighbors or your church will step in to help you get through your crisis season and also the time it takes to recover. Depending on your own personality and that of those who want to help (see *You're Sick They're Not* for why different personalities react differently to crisis), you may or may not want to extend your crisis plan to include who you would prefer to do what.

The most important aspect of that is choosing a Field & Shield person. This is your advocate. They field the curious questions, phone calls, and offers to help, and shield you from the people and things that would drain you of strength.

Your advocate would be the one to update people via phone or social media, tell people when it's a tough day and you're not up for visitors, answer the "What happened?" question for the fifty-ninth time, and let people know your needs if they want to help.

The value of a good Field & Shield friend is beyond words. I hope you have one, or God sends you one soon.

Another person who is great to have in your corner is an Opposite-Brain friend. If you're a right-brain, detail-oriented person, you need someone who sees the big picture, and vice versa. Whenever possible, this friend should come along for important doctor visits, because they will pick up things and remember things you won't.

My Opposite-Brain friend is my husband, Brian. Recently, I went to a neurological surgeon to see if I should get some of my neck bones fused. It was a hefty concept and naturally evoked emotions as I waited in the appointment room. When the doctor arrived, I listened, asked questions, and left feeling a certain way about what I had been told. When I discussed it afterward with Brian, who had come with me, he shared a totally different takeaway from the same meeting. My insecurities about how the doctor might view my odd situation had filtered his response and influenced my understanding of it. Brian was able to reroute the information for me through his logic-based filter, and because of him, I was able to see the doctor's conclusion as a positive step forward instead of the negative way I had seen it.

Be merciful to me, O God, be merciful to me!
For my soul trusts in You; and in the shadow of Your wings
I will make my refuge,
until these calamities have passed by.
Psalm 57:1

Practical Page:

Though all of the following will not always be possible or applicable, here are some practical tips from people who have been through health crisis seasons and want to help you get through yours:

ER or Initial Crisis:
1.   Once you decide to go, don't second guess. It's a waste of energy.
2.   Carry a typed list of your medications in your purse to hand over when asked.
3.   Forgive and let go – everyone will make mistakes including you.

Hospitalization:
1.   Don't feel guilty that you're not getting work done or keeping up with people, etc. Give your body and your spirit permission to rest. It is essential for real healing.
2.   Enjoy the obvious validation of being admitted.
3.   Keep a log – time gets fuzzy and on meds, memory can't be trusted.
4.   Don't expect productivity. Let yourself be sick.

Surgery:
1.   Admit if you're scared.
2.   Ask for prayer. Pray right there together.
3.   Prepare ahead – have Bible verses to focus on or music to listen to, things to help your mind stay on what is true and good and lovely.

<u>Recovery:</u>
1.   Let people help you.
2.   Don't jump back in too quickly and push yourself into another crisis.
3.   Have the goal of a little improvement every day, and let the little be enough.
4.   Funny stuff is worth the money.
5.   Have productive things ready to do for those small bursts of energy that hopefully will come more and more frequently over time.
6.   Whenever it's possible, avoid stress. Be okay with shutting down, turning off the phone and computer, avoiding the news, and telling people you'll update them/get to that/get together/etc. when you're feeling better.

Minor surgery
is an operation performed
on somebody else.
Anonymous

Bad

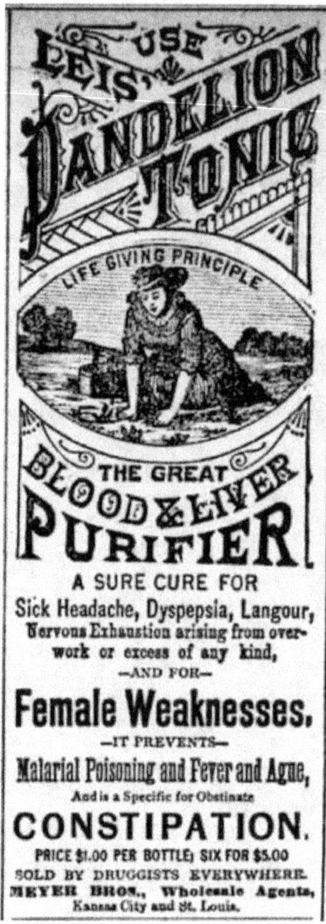

Wow, a "sure cure" for languor, malaria, female
weakness, and constipation all in one.
Why do you suppose it's not still for sale by
"druggists everywhere"?

Worse

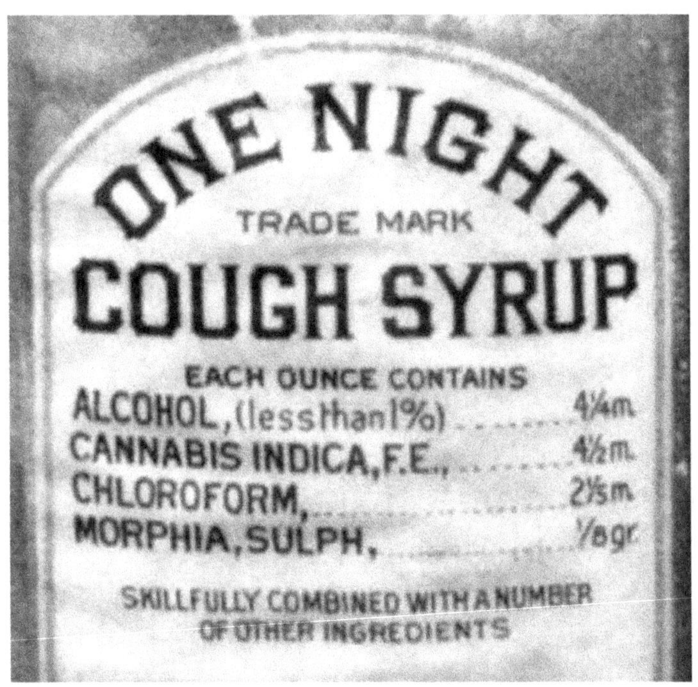

The Federal Food, Drug and Cosmetics Act, making
the sale of addictive drugs illegal over the counter,
was enacted in 1938. Now I know why!

Introducing…

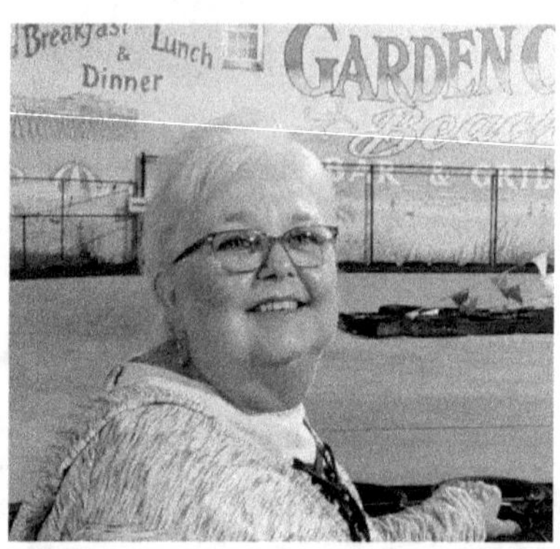

Anita has Myasthenia Gravis, and MuSK antibodies, and calls Prednisone "Satan's TicTacs!"

Her first symptom was double vision, "which I told no one about for several weeks. But one morning I could not hold my head up. It felt like a giant hand was pressing down on the back of my head. I could prop my head up with my hand, but I did not have the muscular strength in my neck and back to hold my head up."

Anita's had her share of side effects. "I am on prednisone which caused me to get glaucoma. The eyedrops I was prescribed to treat the glaucoma have given me absolutely gorgeous long lush eyelashes!"

She's also had her share of difficult medical experiences. "The hospital neuros 'fired me' as a patient because we asked too many questions that they didn't want to answer. That's a long story." Anita shares that, "I find great support in MG support groups! I belong to several online groups via Facebook and feel free to ask questions and share. I also attend a local in-person group once a month."

<u>Her tips for those sick or in pain:</u>
1. A Roomba vacuum cleaner is my best friend.
2. It's OK to say NO, I can't do this today. You don't have to provide a reason or excuse.
3. Keep a gratitude journal. Try to find 3 things every day that either make you smile, or that you are grateful for.

<u>Something someone said that helped:</u>
You are still YOU. You are NOT that disease.
Pajama Days are better than sliced bread with jelly!

O God, You are my God;
early will I seek You;
my soul thirsts for You;
my flesh longs for You
in a dry and thirsty land
where there is no water.
Psalm 63:1

CHAPTER SIX

SARAH'S STORY

If you think nothing is impossible,
try slamming a revolving door.
Anonymous[xii]

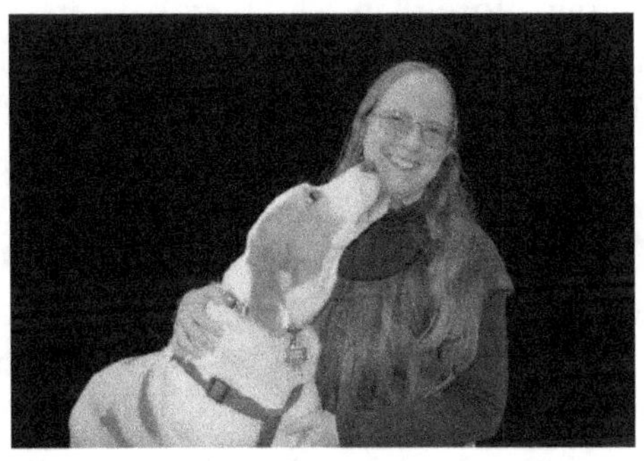

"But you don't look sick." I've heard that hundreds of times, whether from doctors or from well-meaning strangers or friends. The reply in my head goes something like: "Why thank you – I work hard to make myself presentable before I leave the house." Usually, I'm able to keep from actually saying that out loud. You see, unless it's a bad day, my chronic illness is invisible. I look normal. The little service dog that follows me everywhere sometimes betrays my secret; but even then, people usually just assume I'm training the dog for someone else.

75

Although many of my conditions are genetic, they didn't start to become noticeable until I was in high school. It started as mysterious, severe pain and muscle spasms for which nobody could find a cause. In college, temporary paralysis and bizarre allergic reactions joined my list of unexplained symptoms. Then cardiac symptoms a few years later. And the list goes on.

It took over ten years of searching, doctors, testing, and personal research to get my first diagnosis (beyond being told everything was all in my head, of course). Now, more than 100 doctors later, my list of diagnoses is too long to remember and I just print out a condensed version for most appointments because the full list would overwhelm the doctor. Ironically, many of my symptoms actually *are* in my head. Literally – they affect my brain.

Almost all of my illnesses are a result of three primary conditions: Ehlers-Danlos Syndrome, Postural Orthostatic Tachycardia Syndrome, and Mast Cell Activation Syndrome. So that makes explaining them easier. But even with that simplicity, I currently have eight diagnoses that fall into the official "rare disease" category. This means that many doctors don't know what my conditions are, let alone how they interact with each other.

There are benefits to some of them, though. I can more-accurately predict upcoming weather than the weather channel can. Why? Because the varying pressures within my skull have turned me into a human barometer!

Also, life is never boring. For example, my earliest diagnosis was "idiopathic anaphylaxis." I earned that one in college by baffling my allergist. One day in the cafeteria, my throat swelled shut when I smelled a sauce. Yet somehow, I could safely *eat* that same sauce as long as I didn't smell it! He was so confused. A decade later, an equally mysterious situation occurred in which my throat swelled completely closed in response to a temperature change of jumping into a lake. By then, there was a name for my disease, and I was fortunate enough to find an allergist willing to learn about it.

Over the years, I've learned to laugh at and have fun with my chronic illnesses. They aren't going away, and being annoyed by them all the time isn't helpful to anyone. I'm more pleasant to be around when I'm not grumpy, and that puts me on the "nice" list with both friends and medical personnel. Plus, I have to admit that there *are* some pretty funny situations that arise.

I mean, how many people do you know who get sunburned *because* they put on sunscreen? Randomly when I wear my safe-for-me sunscreen, I end up with chemical burns from it. Bright red burns that look like a severe sunburn. When this happens, people usually thoughtfully let me know that I'm getting sunburned and suggest I reapply sunscreen. I don't normally have the heart to tell them that it's actually my sunscreen that did this to me, and that if I hadn't put any on, then I wouldn't be burned! The best part is that the burn stays bright red for weeks.

Or how about the embarrassingly funny things that happen with a service dog tagging along all the time? The first time I took my service dog with me to the dentist, he was well-behaved but young. I took a long-lasting chew treat and a short leash that I could clip to my belt so that he couldn't walk more than six inches from where I told him to stay. He did fantastic for the cleaning and everything went surprisingly smoothly...until the dentist came in and began examining my teeth. Thirty seconds later, I felt a jerk on the leash, followed by the unmistakable sound of my puppy pouncing (yes, like a cat -- I promise you that he's a dog!). I pretended to ignore it. After all, he was a well-trained service dog and the dentist needed me to remain still. Surely nobody would notice. Then another, stronger jerk, a pounce, and claws digging incessantly on the tile floor. Unable to maintain his composure any longer, the dentist started laughing. Another jerk on the leash. I looked down to see what was happening. There was my service dog, supposedly "working," but entirely engrossed in chasing the light from the dentist's headlamp all over the floor. Four years later, my dentist still remembers my complicated medical history every time I walk into his office, and it's all thanks to my service dog choosing to take an unapproved play break.

And yes, my service dog still knows that he will get to play with the dentist and his headlamp at the end of the appointment.

I also do things intentionally to have some fun with my illnesses, and to try to make the best of bad situations. For a while, I had to wear a hard cervical-collar all day every day, which, of course, resulted in a myriad of questions from coworkers and friends. I planned answers in advance, so that I could laugh about it and so that it wouldn't hurt me as much to try to explain repeatedly the real (and scary) reason I was wearing the c-collar. My favorite responses (and both absolutely true!) were: "Oh, my brain is just too big and heavy for my neck to hold up," and "My brain is trying to slide down and escape out my spine, so this keeps it in place!"

Through these years, community has become increasingly important to me. Talking with others with chronic illness not only gives me ideas of things that might help make my life easier, but it also provides perspective and an understanding of what life could be. There's an instant sense of companionship when talking with someone who just "gets it" and doesn't require the explanations of what it means when you say something like, "I'm tired."

Likewise, I'm grateful that God enables us to comfort and encourage one another with the comfort we've received from Him. Years ago, I was alone with my chronic illness (didn't even know the term, let alone anyone else who struggled with it!) and I clung to the hope that one day God would use my unexplained and mysterious suffering to encourage someone else. I clung to that prayer for almost fifteen years, never seeing fruit but learning to endure and persevere because His Word says He's good and He has worthwhile purposes that I don't always see. In the last three years, I've had the unbelievable blessing of seeing bushels of fruit. Lives that have literally been saved because I was in the right place at the right time with the right medical training and personal experience. Lives that have been completely changed because I took the time to listen and put mysterious pieces together that no doctor had been able to. People who have been encouraged because finally somebody believed them *and* could help them make daily life more manageable. It's such a blessing and encouragement to see those fifteen lonely years used by Him!

The joy of the Lord is your strength.
Nehemiah 8:10c

Practical Page:

Sarah's Tips:

Learn to laugh.
Frequently. Whether at your own body/situation, the goofy antics of a pet, or a silly TV show or meme. Laughing really does help, both physically with reducing pain and mentally/emotionally with the day-to-day reality of chronic illness.

Assume positive intent.
Honestly, this choice has been a life-changer for me. It's so easy to just assume that the doctor didn't remember details about me because he doesn't really care about me, that the ER didn't *really* want to help me, that my friends have forgotten all about me because nobody checks in anymore or invites me out, etc. Most of the time, those things aren't anywhere close to true. It's also really easy to do this with God, feeling like He must be punishing me or must not love me because He allows all these bad things to happen. That for sure isn't true – God neither delights in nor wastes our suffering. He suffers along with us. Repeating to my heart and mind to assume positive intent has helped keep me from a lot of bitterness that would otherwise consume my life.

Find community.
If you have access to local support groups or others with chronic illness, awesome! If you don't, there are quite a few now online. (Just be careful – online

support groups in particular can be wearisome or increase anxiety as well.) I also encourage you to create your own local community – help your friends understand what chronic illness life is like, little by little, and to point them to Jesus during it. Not all friends will understand, but those few who do become precious companions in life.

83

If we shouldn't eat at night,
why is there a light in the fridge?

Anonymous[xiii]

Bad

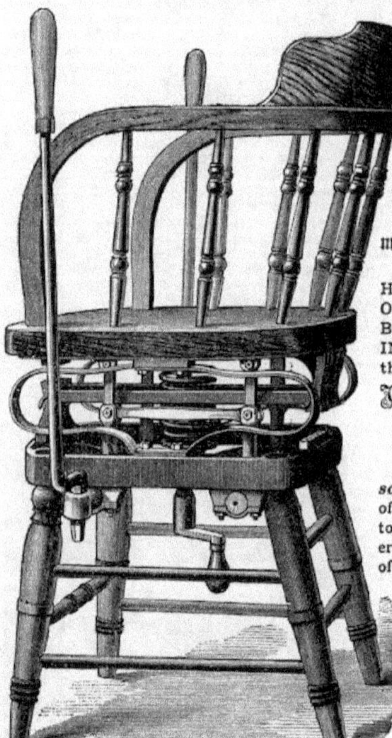

A great relief if your saddle-horse is taking up
too much room in your home.

Worse

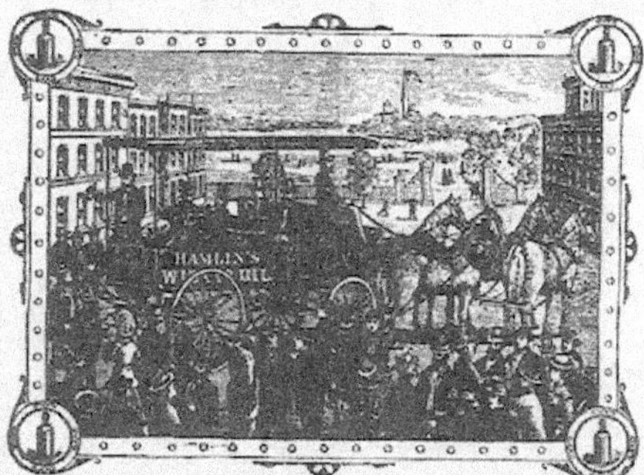

Is it made out of wizards?

Introducing…

Jacqueline has Rheumatoid Arthritis. When asked if she looks sick, she responded, "Nope. Healthy as a horse."

She got diagnosed ten years ago. "When I'm quiet you know pain is too much. I do try and be real. If you ask I will tell you I am hurting. I rarely tell anyone my disease because the 'instant cures' I have heard are insane!"

<u>Who do you like to get advice from?</u>
Doctor who practices natural and traditional. They are hard to find but they are out there.

<u>What is a weird symptom you've had?</u>
I cannot lay on my ears. Yep. It's weird. I have cut holes in my expensive foam pillow that are just a bit bigger than my ears. I am a side sleeper, so I have two holes in my pillow. One for each side.

<u>Does it help talking with others with same issues or not?</u>
It did at first. I wanted to learn about my illness. I quickly realized "healthy" people did not realize, understand, or downplayed how horribly I felt. So I went to RA websites. At first I was in tears that these people get me! After a while though, most sites just really bummed me out. They pulled me down more than I was pulling down myself.

Jacqueline's tips:
If I ever find a new RA buddy, I try and be an encourager and a listening ear. I tell them one, and only one, website that I feel tells them a lot. I do not talk about the really depressing stuff with my new buddy unless they ask.

Anything else?
Make sure you are resting during the day.
Realize you need to take things a little slower if you are going to interact with family later on that night.
It's not your fault you are sick.

When the poor and needy seek water,
and there is none,
and their tongue faileth for thirst,
I the Lord will hear them,
I the God of Israel will not forsake them.
Isaiah 41:17 KJV

CHAPTER SEVEN

AS BAD AS IT GETS

When I cannot read, when I cannot think,
when I cannot even pray, I can trust.
J. Hudson Taylor[xiv]

The day I was admitted into a hospital for the first time was, I'm pretty sure, the worst of my life to that point. We had been traveling. I'd had a cold for a couple of weeks that I could not shake. As we drove down from Ohio to Georgia with plans to leave soon for Indonesia, I definitely felt worse.

It had been in the plan to stop at a special place halfway through the trip, but I couldn't enjoy the atmosphere or the amazing food. It was memorable in the worst way that I got the most expensive dinner I've ever had, took two bites, and threw up.

I was up all that night sick, with so much pain in my left side and shoulder I couldn't lay on that side. It started hurting just to breathe.

The next morning my husband took me to a clinic, where I feared hearing I was overreacting and merely had a bad cold. It was a relief to hear the doctor say I had pneumonia. At least that gave validation to the fact that I felt so miserable. He said I should get checked into a hospital, but we still had a four-hour drive ahead of us, so he gave me a shot that was supposed to take away the pain and off we went.

The shot didn't work. I sat in the back with my toddler, crying over every bump, every jolt. It was a very long trip.

Finally, finally, we got to the ER near my parents' house. I was beyond relieved, until we got inside and found out they were filled up and there were people waiting and we would have to wait too. (If I had known then what I know now, I'd have gotten right back in that car and gone to a better hospital, but we figured it was the ER, you know, emergency, so they'd get to me very soon.)

Those next four hours were among the most painful of my life. Every breath I took hurt. Other people in the ER looked at me and then away in sympathy. My dad came, stayed for awhile, then left with tears in his eyes. Brian, my husband, stayed with me, but there really wasn't anything he could do.

I wanted someone to storm in and convince these people that I needed help. Finally they called me back, asked questions, checked my x-rays, noted that I had pneumonia, then send me back into the waiting room. I guess I didn't impress them enough. Had I been able to tell them what I found out later—that I also had pleurisy, bacterima, and empyema, maybe that would have helped. If only, right?

When they did eventually get to me, the doctor gave me a shot of the most powerful pain-killer they had. It took care of some of the pain, but I still hurt so much I couldn't lay down.

By nighttime, I was put into a room far at the end of the ER because they had no available beds up in the hospital so I couldn't be officially admitted. As I mentioned in another book, this was the room for mentally unstable patients. It didn't even have a call button. I waited for hours for pain meds. I even walked out into the hallway to get someone's attention once.

Finally, I think it was sometime the next day, Brian became my knight in shining armor by finding some PR guy in the hospital and explaining our unpleasant situation. After that they were going to move me up into the regular hospital so I'd get better care, but then they had a glitch because the doctor had never ordered me admitted into the mental room, so they couldn't discharge me from it since I wasn't supposed to be there in the first place. Eventually they did get me to a room, where a host of other misadventures waited for me, and after a lifesaving surgery and nine days in ICU, I got to go home and recover from the whole ordeal.

Don't you feel sorry for me? As my grandpa used to say, "That'll get you in the gizzard."

This is the part where I'm supposed to complain about the system. How laws need to be changed. How we deserve better treatment. How the world owes us something.

If that's what you're hoping for, you picked the wrong book. It's not going to happen.

Why not?

Because I know too much about how good we have it. I've lived in places where the average medical care is horrifying. I've seen beggars with massive tumors stretching out their necks and permanently tilting their heads toward the side because they cannot afford even the basest of care. I've heard about patients so poor they sold the medication they were given, to feed their families. I've known about people dying because of treatment based on superstition, or religion, or just culture.

If you ever want to think we have it bad, study Chinese foot binding. For hundreds and likely thousands of years, over a billion young Chinese girls, usually starting around the age of five, had their feet made as tiny as possible. Older women, including the girl's mother, would fold all their toes except the one big toe under their feet, and then bind them with wet bandages so that when the bandages dried, they tightened until each toe broke, then the arch of the foot broke. These children were forced to walk on the huge wounds their feet had become to make them break more quickly. Enduring this suffering was necessary if they were to have husbands and honor their families. One out of ten died from it.

I could tell you stories that would curl your insides, like the day I touched a woman lying on the street only to realize she was already dead, but I will spare your heart things I wish I did not know. Because of where I have been and what I have seen, I will not be one of those people who rants about how the system needs to change. Yes, people make mistakes. Yes, sometimes they are not as caring as they should be.

They are human. I won't say I didn't experience anger and frustration and disappointment over my medical care many times, emphasis on the many part, but when I think about the fact that everything above hell itself is grace from God, I know that I have already been given more than abundance. Every moment without pain is a gift. The fact that I was born into this great country where I am free to go to a doctor, have enough money to buy medicine, and have the option of researching and gaining knowledge—these things are all great gifts.

Perhaps sometimes experiencing long waits or unexpected bills or cranky caregivers has helped me be more compassionate to those who are treated that way all the time because of their gender or their race or their income level. I have only experienced a tiny glimpse of the life they live every day.

Perhaps sometimes we are sent into the medical world not so much for our own benefit, but so we can be a blessing to someone else there in need. Maybe to a nurse whose life is falling apart, and she can't fake a smile that day. Maybe to a fellow patient who never has any visitors. Maybe to a family member in a waiting room who's just heard the worst news and doesn't know where to turn.

Remember the book where I talked about how everything good comes from God? That hospital was the place I learned that, and I learned something else along with it.

I have the opportunity to be that good thing to others. To be God's gift to them. When something would go wrong, my response was either from my flesh (irritation, fear, anger) or from God (me allowing Him to fill me with His grace and then show it to others). My actions and reactions always fell into one of those two categories. Either the bad in the world that's to be expected from humanity, or a good thing which reflects God's presence in this world and in His children.

The knowledge sobered me, because frankly, I didn't feel like I needed to be responsible for my reactions in that setting. I was being mistreated. It wasn't fair. I had come there to be helped, not to have to minister to others.

God's whisper has stayed with me. People who do not know Him have very few resources for having the right attitude and doing the right thing. I should stop expecting them to act like people who have God's strength. I, however, do have that grace to help in time of need.

So who is the one who needs the most care? I might be suffering now physically, but that nurse might be living the pain of spiritual emptiness and lack of hope. I'm wanting her to set aside her own issues to minister to me, but maybe it should be the other way around.

That's extremely not fun when in pain, I know. But I also know that during those fifteen days in the hospital, the times when I was feeling more stable, a little better, that's when God would send the difficult people my way. When I was struggling and could not take it anymore, God would send me caring nurses, often Christian ones, who were a blessing. My ICU nurse held my hand during the worst moments, and even offered to pay for my husband to fly back to the US to be with me. What a precious gift her kindness was.

I doubt I was a blazing light of grace in that hospital. I would love to be able to say I ministered to others in my need, but I didn't. I learned good lessons for the future though, including what some wise person once said, "Some days the victory is just in enduring."

Enduring makes us strong. And though I hope and pray there will never be a follow-up of that whole experience, if God chooses that for me, may He give me enough grace to give grace to others.

May He do the same for you.

I will open rivers in high places, and fountains in the midst of the valleys: I will make the wilderness a pool of water, and the dry land springs of water.
Isaiah 41:18 KJV

Practical Page:

Express Gratitude Instead of Guilt

"I'm sorry you had to do all of this so I could come."
"I feel badly you had to work so hard on my account."

The above often unintentionally require a response of reassurance and possibly a minimizing of the other person's efforts to make us feel better.
Unfortunately, those responses often make us feel worse instead, because they now have put their own effort down when we know it was costly for them.

Try:

"I could not have come if you hadn't done all this extra work for me. Thank you."
"It means so much to me to be here. I appreciate all you did to make it possible."

These lift up the person and their effort. They recognize our acceptance of the gift they have given with their time and actions, and offer appreciation rather than an indirect request for even more effort through additional reassurance.

Receiving a gift of help with gratitude rather than guilt leaves both parties happier in the end.

The human body experiences
a powerful gravitational pull
in the direction of hope.
That is why the patient's hopes
are the physician's secret weapon.
They are the hidden ingredients
in any prescription.

Norman Cousins[xv]

Bad

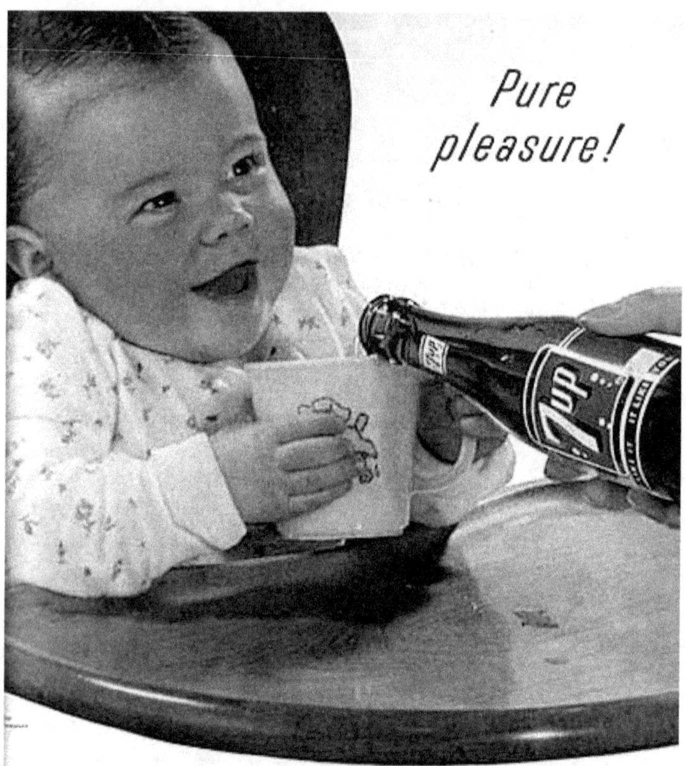

Pure. Wholesome. Seriously?

Worse

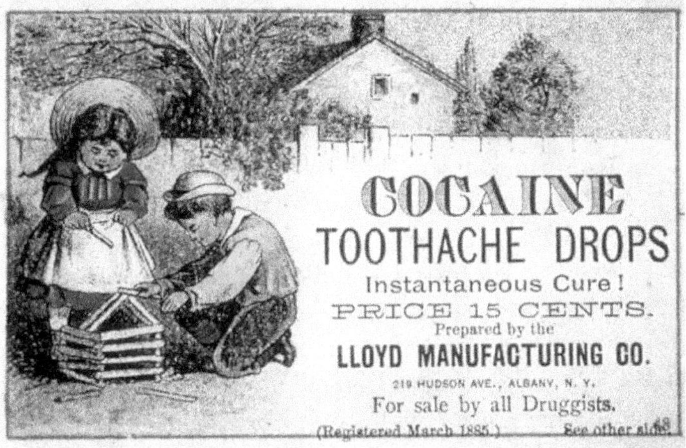

Who thought this was a good idea?
Freaking out right now on behalf
of all those poor kids.

Introducing…

Laura K. has seen close to one hundred doctors. Her list of illnesses includes adrenal insufficiency, juvenile rheumatoid arthritis, fibromyalgia, "which means we don't know why you hurt," idiopathic gastroparesis, POTS, and glaucoma.

Laura has extremely interesting symptoms and side effects, including, "a really quick drop in blood pressure making me look like I'm drunk. I can't see straight or walk straight until my vision clears and my BP regulates. I also have a blind eye and all my eye doctors know it, but I think it's hilarious when they hand me the eye patch to cover the blind eye to read the eye chart. Night terrors about spiders have made me scream so loudly I literally woke up the neighbor who came outside with a cast iron skillet!"

And that's not all. "I dislocated my hip out the back (posteriorly) after I had an anterior front hip replacement. It has never been done or seen before in the hospital I was in or with my surgeon. I also begin to talk out of my head completely nonsensically when I don't have enough prednisone and something is wrong with my body. I can say some pretty funny things and have zero memory of it later. My stomach swells and it looks like I am nine months pregnant when my GP is acting up and my food isn't being digested, but I have been asked when the baby is due. Since I had to have a hysterectomy and have black adopted kids when I am white, that turns kind of funny."

Does it help talking with others with the same issues or not?

Yes, very much so. I know I'm not crazy. Otherwise I begin to think I have a mental problem not a physical one. Even though even with the oddest combination of symptoms they normally find a cause, it just takes a LONG time.

What's something someone said that helped you?

That I matter. Even with all my illness and problems, I still matter.

Laura K's tip:

Accept your limitations. Do what you can to give yourself a quality of life. If it means doing nothing until your family is home and with you, do nothing so you can enjoy family. Asking for help with cleaning and laundry and such is not saying anything about your character, it is giving you time to spend with your loved ones in the brief windows you have while feeling somewhat better.

You are My servant,
I have chosen you
and have not cast you away.
Isaiah 41:9b

CHAPTER EIGHT

TO CHURCH OR NOT TO CHURCH

*Have you ever noticed that anybody
driving slower than you is an idiot,
and anyone going faster than you is a maniac?*
George Carlin[xvi]

It's hard to explain to a healthy person how exhausting getting ready for church can be. The best parallel I can think of is getting an eighteen-month-old toddler ready for church. You have this great little dress, an adorable hairstyle in mind, sweet little shoes, and socks with ruffles.

Reality barges in with a diaper change, breakfast, face and body cleanup from bites that did not make it to the mouth, then the attempt to restrain the wiggles enough to get the dress on and secured. After that is the meltdown over the wrong bow or wrong whatever, giving up on the adorable shoes for ones you can get on before she wanders off, plus at least three other random distractions. In the end, she looks cherubic, and you're a wreck. You carry her to the car muttering that next week you're taking her to church in her pajamas and bare feet.

That's how it can be for us. Most of us don't wear diapers (yet), and don't wiggle when getting dressed (unless something's a size too small), but that feeling at the end is on target. We may look ready for church

103

but we feel ready for bed. Our exhaustion is not because we get distracted by outside things, but our bodies are just so busy fighting their inner war, and sending us messages that it has bigger priorities than us looking put together, messages like fatigue and cold sweats, or dizziness and nausea, or needing to take extra medication that turns us into mental zombies, etc.

When we finally are ready, we often don't have any energy left for the drive there, much less sitting, often with pain, in an upright position for an hour or more. And then there's the talking. Do you feel snob guilt? I have such a hard time admitting that talking with people is draining. Really draining. It's not that I don't like people. It's just that if you have nothing left to give, being personable is like someone handing that beautifully dressed child back to you between services and saying, "She undressed herself and needs a diaper change. Can you take care of that before the next service starts?"

And then, after all that overexertion, someone tells us cheerfully, "Well, you don't look sick!" They mean it in the best way possible, but it sometimes sounds like, "Well, you must be faking it." We are faking it, but not being sick. We're faking being well. In that arena, we can succeed to our detriment.

There was a season when chronic pain added so much to my church experience it was comical...almost. My Ehlers-Danlos syndrome plus scoliosis causes pain, and church pews seem especially created to cause as much back discomfort as possible. (Way back, some thought the less comfortable you were, the more spiritual you were. There's some validity in that—if we all put our feet up and wore yoga pants while eating Cheetos through the service, we might not be paying as much attention. Plus, people in yoga pants with their feet up smacking on Cheetos would drive a lot of us to a different denomination to avoid the visual.) If I did make it to Sunday school, which was rare, I had to rush out to my vehicle between services and eat a specially chosen snack to keep my blood sugar stable through the main service. I'd get back in and get settled on our pew, then set up my paraphernalia. I'd open the fold-up footstool brought from home so I could partially prop my feet up (no yoga pants if you were worried, but sometimes I did wear floor-length flowy skirts so I could curl my legs up onto the pew without being uncouth). Then I'd get my doggie ball out of my purse. It was really a doggie ball, one of those dense, throw toys from a dollar store. I kept one in the car, one at home and one extra. That went under my left hip to mash the fascia and help with the pain, and also to make my hips more level. It's a good thing I had given up choir at this point due to my asthma. The doggie ball might have earned questioning looks if the polka-dot footstool didn't. Then there was my inhaler if someone who smelled nice happened to hug me, plus pain pills, antihistamines, blood sugar meds, and a few others for odd conditions, plus sometimes a bottle of water to take such pills when needed, hopefully during a transition so I wouldn't be a distraction. Also were the cough drops and Big Red for nausea or lung irritation, and maybe a bit of sugar in case it was needed.

Some days I wished I had kept my kids' diaper bags to hold everything.

I grew up in a culture where you were at church anytime the doors were open. I went to a Christian college that required chapel four times a week along with the four required Sunday and Wednesday services. So…

Choosing to stay home can be laden with guilt. Choosing to go can be laden with pain. What's a girl to do?

Here's my question for whether or not to go through all it takes to go to church: Which one brings you closer to God? Now, this is not one of those blanket statements that means you can quit church because you can worship Him just as well at home. We need family, the family of God even more than biological family. I'm not saying skip that just because it takes more for us to be there than some others. However, there are times when it's clearly not possible. Other times it could be done, but it would take everything we have to show up and be able to be nice to people, which makes it not about God or growing in His Word, but rather about faking it. Sometimes, I personally believe that what I need most is some quiet time by myself with the Lord. When the kids were little especially, that set apart time was hard to come by, and I valued it. I still do.

Make church time a time to draw closer to your Savior, whether that means going for the usual reasons, or perhaps going with the recognition you'll be ministering to others so it's worth sacrifice, or staying home and having a talk with Jesus and hearing from Him through His Word.

The goal is to know Him and enjoy Him, not to put on a show—not a big collective show or a small one-person faking it show either. Church shouldn't be about us. It should be about God.

So what does God want for you this Sunday?

Rejoice always, pray without ceasing,
in everything give thanks;
for this is the will of God in Christ Jesus for you.
1 Thessalonians 5:16-18

Practical Page:

<u>If you ask, people will likely come up with three optional answers for the big church question:</u>
1.   You're fine. You should go.
2.   You're not fine but could still go, so you should.
3.   You're sick or in the hospital and should stay in bed.

<u>There are actually six options, at least:</u>
1.   You're fine, so you go.
2.   You're not fine, but can and do go, and it's good. You're glad you went.
3.   You're not fine and shouldn't go, but you push yourself and go anyway. It's bad, and you pay for it the next several hours/days.
4.   You're not fine and don't go, but you should have. Feel guilty and regretful.
5.   You're not fine and shouldn't go and don't. You feel refreshed by time alone with God, or enjoy a sermon via radio or TV.
6.   You're not fine and not sure if you should go or not. This is probably the most common. If you go, you might regret it. If you don't go, you might regret it. I have zero advice for this because it's my big struggle too.

What do you think? Have you ever asked God about your Sunday choice? This next Sunday, maybe you should.

I wish I was a kid again
so everyone would be proud of me
for taking a long nap.
Anonymous[xvii]

Bad

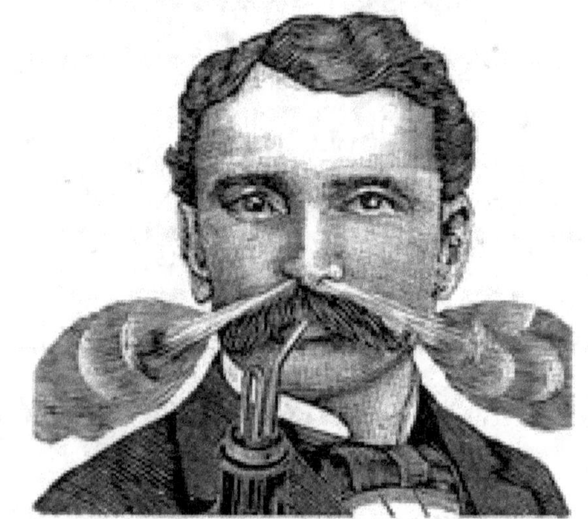

Do you have to have a mustache for it to work?

Worse

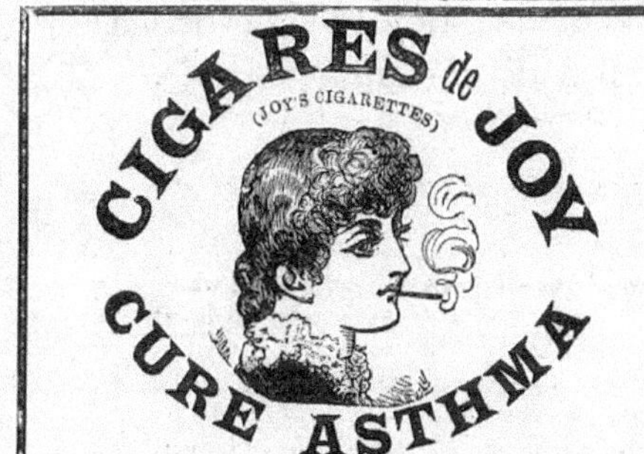

All this time I should have been
smoking to fix my asthma?
Apparently "the most eminent physicians
and medical authors" think so.

Introducing…

Tanya has fibromyalgia and chronic fatigue syndrome. She gets chest pain and feels like she's standing on her head and all the blood is rushing to it.

She does have friends online, "but it would be nice if I had some in-person friends who understand."

<u>Tanya's advice:</u>
It's okay to ask for help.
Healing is a process and multifaceted.

For which of you,
intending to build a tower,
does not sit down first
and count the cost,
whether he has enough to finish it?
Luke 14:28

CHAPTER NINE

COST VERSUS BENEFIT

Take my advice. I'm not using it.
David J. Henderhand[xviii]

An opportunity came up for me to basically have a free trip to Florida by tagging along to a conference my husband needed to attend. It was close to St. Augustine, a special place I used to visit as a little girl. I have such happy memories from the Veteran's Day parade, of people saluting my dad in his Navy whites, of the strange oddities in the Ripley's museum, of the unwritten stories buried beneath old, weathered gravestones.

I wanted to show my children the amazing historical sites, and of course, see the ocean again.

Even considering going was a big deal. Two years ago we had taken what I expected to be my last trip before I accepted my spiral toward disability due to chronic pain and illness. Then brain surgery made a major difference in my pain and also took away several of my "diseases" that had really been caused by Chiari Malformation, i.e. my brain being too big for my skull.

That's a story for another book.

The surgery relieved a lifetime of compression in my spinal canal and made a vast improvement in nearly every arena of illness except my asthma, which has since gotten worse. I'm more sensitive to triggers than ever, so while the possibility of the trip was exciting, it would not be without cost or risk.

We talked and prayed over the options, the possibilities good and bad, and whether or not it was worth the cost and risk.

With that nervous, hesitant excitement I'm sure you're familiar with, we decided to go…

Prepping for the Possibilities

We had a family meeting before the trip about expectations and the need for everyone to invest to make it possible. I know, it leeches some of the fun out of it, but it would leech a lot more if we ended up in the ER, or had to leave early and had devastated kids because we hadn't approached the possibilities and needs.

My children were told up front that I really, really wanted to go, but it depended on my lungs and the hotels and such, so even if we could go, it wasn't certain we could stay.

With the acceptance of that prerequisite, making this work was a team effort and removed my usual dread of things going wrong and "me" ruining everyone's fun. Our family prayed about this trip for weeks, so all of us saw the small victories as gifts from God and this entire trip, each continued day, as His answer to our prayers. Putting the whole thing in our Heavenly Father's hands put the length and abilities under His jurisdiction and out of mine. We all invested and worked to make it succeed, but ultimately it was up to the Lord's will.

Thoughts from the Final Day of the Trip

I'm sitting in my van, my safe breathing space, with a gorgeous view beyond the parking lot of gentle ocean waves lapping against the walls of the old fort in St. Augustine, Florida. At this point, my lungs are so flared, the inevitability of a smoker or person with perfume passing by were I to go walking around outside, and the instant misery that would cause, keeps me from feeling sorry for myself in my bubble.

I'm choosing to view this as a successful trip. The hotels were rough, but not so bad I had to sneak out to sleep in the van. I had to wear my mask almost the entire trip, but we didn't have to come home early. The ocean was a wonderful gift, and with the added joy of watching my family play in it, made all of this worth it. Even now on this last stop before we head home, I may brave emerging from my bubble to walk the exterior of the fort and catch a little of that gloriously salty sea air, with the hopes that no one who smells will get within twenty feet.

We who live with illness and limitation can't ever expect a perfectly smooth trip, any more than a person on a limited budget can spend lavishly on a vacation without any thought for money.

That's a good analogy. Let's chase it.

Say you want to go on a wonderful trip. You have $200. Your choices are either to fit what you do, where you go, and how long you stay into that limit of $200, or you'll need to come up with more money to spend. Jumping in the car with $200 and going on your whims and hoping it will all work out would be foolish. People who do that dig deep holes of debt that will catch up to them with major negative consequences.

It is the same with us. We have only so much physically to spend, so we can't be spontaneous and hope our bodies hold up without any issues. I'm a natural optimist, and dislike having to think through all the possible bad things that might happen, but trust me, it's way better than spending the vacation in Urgent Care.

For me these days, "vacations" just aren't worth it. The extra pain and extra meds required, plus the—you get it so I'll skip the explanation of all that—makes the cost not worth the benefit. Right now while I'm in a stuck place waiting for insurance to approve trying a med made from Chinese hamster ovaries of all things, I'm so unstable that if things don't change I'll probably miss out on Thanksgiving and Christmas get-togethers this year. I'll be in my safely protected home, my bubble, because going outside it this year is just too much.

This trip I'm on right now was worth the risk and cost. My kids are growing up quickly. Coming here with them was important to me. It wasn't a healthy choice for my body, but my body is not always the highest priority. These past three days, they have been my priority, which is why I'm sitting in the van as I write this, missing out, and it's okay. I enjoyed multiple wonderful moments of laughter and love and sharing memories. Those will be precious to me long after the physical ramifications from this trip have settled.

We do have to make allowances and boundaries for our illnesses. But I refuse to let them steal my life. I don't want to just exist, waiting to feel better. I want to live.

Therefore, on goes my mask, and I'm off to look at the sea and marvel at the gift today is.

P.S. I got to sit outside for over half an hour, twice, and God cleared the area for me almost entirely. I saw a turtle and a crab, and flopping fish, and got sunburnt enjoying the goodness of God through His beauty. It doesn't always work that way, but today it did, and I'm thankful.

Practical Page:

Special events are not a vacation for us. Rather than a getaway from our stressors, they tend to inflame them and require extra work instead of offering a break.

Back to that budget analogy, impulse buyers can spend too much and regret some of their choices. Non-spenders can hold back so much they are missing out. The challenge, as in so much of life, is to find a good balance.

Make Purposeful Choices
That great view outside I mentioned is lovely and draws me to come nearer the water and sunshine. The fort edge bordering the water is a hard concrete-type surface. No soft benches would mean pain later in the day for my Ehlers-Danlos Syndrome. If I decide the cost is worth the benefit, then in a few hours when I'm aching, I can accept that because I chose to spend that. If I didn't choose, I'm likely to complain or feel sorry for myself that other people can sit and watch the water, but I can't…whine, whimper, sigh.
Nobody likes that, not even me.

Expect to need a Break after the "Break"
Also, recognize and accept that you will need time to recover from special times. Make the habit of scheduling time afterward and then take it, without a shred of guilt.
Not
One
Shred.

Stop worrying about
the world ending today.
It's already tomorrow in Australia.
Charles M. Schulz[xix]

Bad

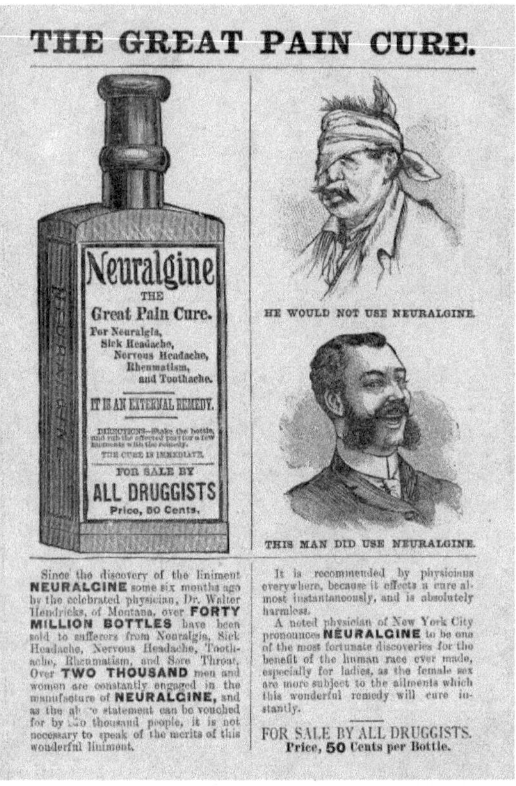

Even back when it was just drawings,
advertisers relied on the power of comparison. Look
how miserable the top guy is compared to the man
who used this "Great Pain Cure,"
who clearly is happy, healthy, and able to grow
a vast amount of facial hair.

Worse

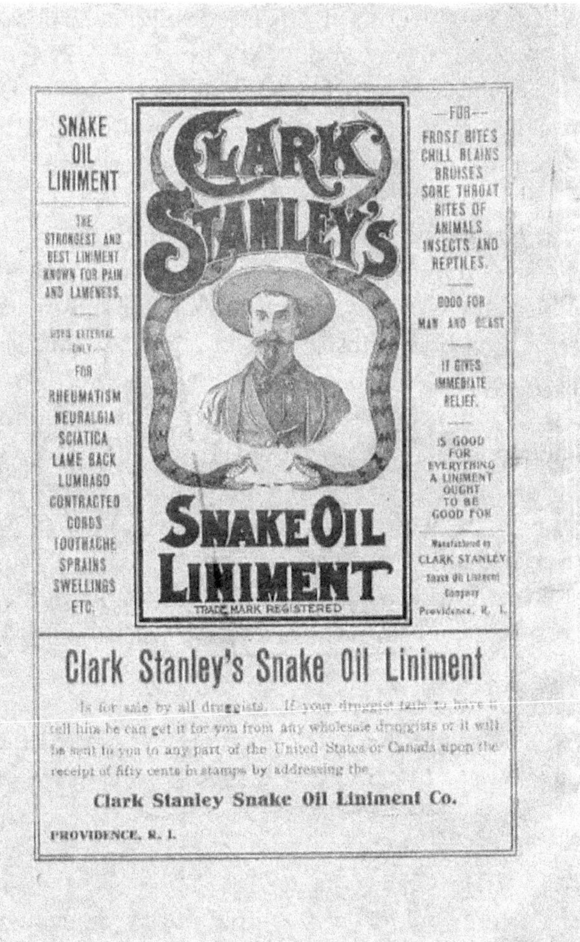

I thought snake oil was only a term!

Introducing…

Marie has had Multiple Sclerosis since 1983. "My best advice has come from my amazing chiropractor who knows more about MS than my PCP. My greatest help comes from listening to audio Bible through earphones. In the last year and a half I have listened to the entire Bible 3 1/2 times through."

What is a weird symptom you've had?
Let's see…Double vision that can split into double-double…Hyperacusis, which is extreme sensitivity to noise…Full-body muscle spasms…My hair felt like it was electric… Numbness from the upper teeth to the scalp…Temporary loss of ability to taste food…to name a few.

What is a weird or funny side effect you've experienced?
I'm now officially allergic to 23 prescription meds.
The oddest side effect was when a combination of Dilaudid and Clinoril prescribed for back pain caused my arms and legs to jerk and flap.
Novocaine (which has epinephrine) has caused me to shake so hard I nearly slid off the dental chair.

Marie's tips:
Ask for help when you need it. Years ago I realized that suffering alone was a point of pride with me. People genuinely wanted to help, but if I didn't tell them what I needed, how could they know? Asking for help is not necessarily a sign of weakness, but a sign of humility. Humility does not come easily to me

as a strong-willed and independent person. I need to allow others to "work out" their gift of serving others. Humbling myself and accepting their service is a blessing to both of us.

<u>Something someone said that helped:</u>
A pastor who visited our church many years ago wrote me a letter. He told me that he believed God has chosen me for Multiple Sclerosis because He knew I was ready, and that God would be given the glory through my suffering. It was a hard concept to understand at the time, but I later understood the depth of what the pastor said.

I have adopted two Scripture passages as my comfort verses:

2 Corinthians 12:9-10
But he said to me, "My grace is sufficient for you, for my power is made perfect in weakness." Therefore I will boast all the more gladly about my weaknesses, so that Christ's power may rest on me. That is why, for Christ's sake, I delight in weaknesses, in insults, in hardships, in persecutions, in difficulties. For when I am weak, then I am strong.

2 Corinthians 1:3-4
Praise be to the God and Father of our Lord Jesus Christ, the Father of compassion and the God of all comfort, who comforts us in all our troubles, so that we can comfort those in any trouble with the comfort we ourselves receive from God.

She opens her mouth with wisdom,
and on her tongue
is the law of kindness.
Prov 31:26

CHAPTER TEN

INDIGNATION OR INSPIRATION

*If things are tough, remember that every flower that
ever bloomed had to go through a whole lot of dirt
to get there. The almighty Father will use life's reverses
to move you forward. So do not keep grieving about a
bitter experience. The present is slipping by while you are
regretting the past and worrying about the future.*
Barbara Johnson[xx]

Three days ago, a dear friend did something
"normal" that has had me flared up ever since. She
had no idea her small action would cause me
suffering, but it did. I've done inhalers and my
nebulizer and ice packs and antihistamines, and blah
blah blah. I finally went to the doctor this morning
for a steroid shot, and will head to the pharmacy for a
prednisone pack. You know the drill.

Unfortunately, irritation is one of the strong,
unwanted symptoms. I did get frustrated. I did vent
to my husband (or perhaps complain might be a more
accurate word). More than being frustrated with her
for not knowing all my triggers, etc., I think I'm just
angry at how fragile I am, at how extensive the
ramifications are for things so insignificant that others
don't even think about them.

I recognize we shouldn't expect everyone to know
about all our quirky needs and be aware of them every
moment. My mother has diabetes, and though I know

what a sugar low feels like, I still can't necessarily recognize when she's spiraling down into one because so much of what is happening is inside her. I have another friend dealing with major food allergies right now, and even though I know that and care, I still didn't catch myself before I offered her a bite of something on her no list.

Even still, when we're in pain, fighting to breathe, or any other number of struggles that can happen from someone else's unwitting actions, it's hard not to feel…hmm, so many words come to mind. Irritated? Resentful? Perhaps even bitter about our limitations or certain people who do not recognize, acknowledge or validate them?

On the way home from the doctor today, I saw a homeless man on the side of the road. Does he have anyone acknowledging or validating his needs and sufferings? I don't know. Kind of makes me think outside my forced self-absorption for a moment.

Bigger than that, however, is something that happened prior to this latest flare. A few weeks ago, on a day when I had to take extra meds and wear my mask to make it through an event, I was talking to a very nice woman whose attention was spread between me and her two special needs children, one sitting on each side of her. She gave them both loving attention at each of their frequent interruptions. I was impressed with her gentle and calm spirit. She has four children total, all still at home.

Her husband died without warning only a year ago.

As I marveled at this woman's gracious spirit despite her incredible suffering, far beyond anything

I've gone through, I tried to offer a bit of sympathy by mentioning the inconsiderate things people can say or do when they don't know what to say or do. In part, I might have brought it up because I myself didn't know what to say or do, but usually when I say this to people with chronic illness, it gives them an opportunity to vent a little, or at least acknowledge that they've been hurt by innocuous comments people did not realize were wounding.

This woman surprised me. She did not take the opportunity. Instead, her response was, "Everybody has something. I know I need a lot of grace, and I need to give grace."

Those words were at the same time convicting and inspiring. I have thought of them often since, including the past few days. I need grace. I need to give grace. Everybody has something.

I can focus on the grace I need, and fuss that people don't understand, or get frustrated that my pain, not being visible, is not believed or taken seriously. Or I can recognize that all those around me are dealing with their own kind of pain or struggle, and theirs may be more invisible, and deeper, than mine.

That's not to say it's wrong to vent sometimes, or express the frustration over our situation. But that shouldn't become our default attitude, a root of bitterness that will grow into a weed of bitterness (and we all know what weeds do).

I want to carry my new friend's words with me, more than just a motto, more like a lifestyle or creed. I need a lot of grace; I need to give grace. Everybody has something.

And I want to be the kind of person whose response and words can inspire others to a higher perspective, as she, in that small moment, inspired me.

When He gives quietness,
who then can make trouble?
Job 34:29

Practical Page:

Take the Debt to the One Who Can Pay

It doesn't feel good to be on the receiving end in an unbalanced way. When it comes to our health needs, however, the imbalance is not one we can fix. This can lead to extra guilt or even an avoidance of the people we feel we owe because being around them makes us feel badly.

This need not be. We know the God who owns all things and supplies His children's needs according to His unlimited resources (Phil. 4:19). If He assigned this person to provide your needs, then He is the One responsible to repay and reward that.

Therefore, we can avoid saying or writing:

"I wish I could pay you back somehow, but..."

"How can I ever repay you for all you did?"

These phrases can cause the helper to say it wasn't a big deal or offer some other automatic reassurance that leaves you feeling even more in their debt.

Now, knowing Who is the source to provide repayment, we can say or write:

"I prayed today that God blesses you for the blessing you have been for me."

"May God repay you for being so kind."

Or simply quote Ruth 2:12: *The* LORD *repay your work, and a full reward be given you by the* LORD *God of Israel, under whose wings you have come for refuge.*

"What kind of work do you do?"
a woman passenger enquired
of the man travelling in her
train compartment.
"I'm a Naval surgeon," he replies.
"My word!" sputtered the woman,
"How you doctors
specialize these days."

xxi

Bad

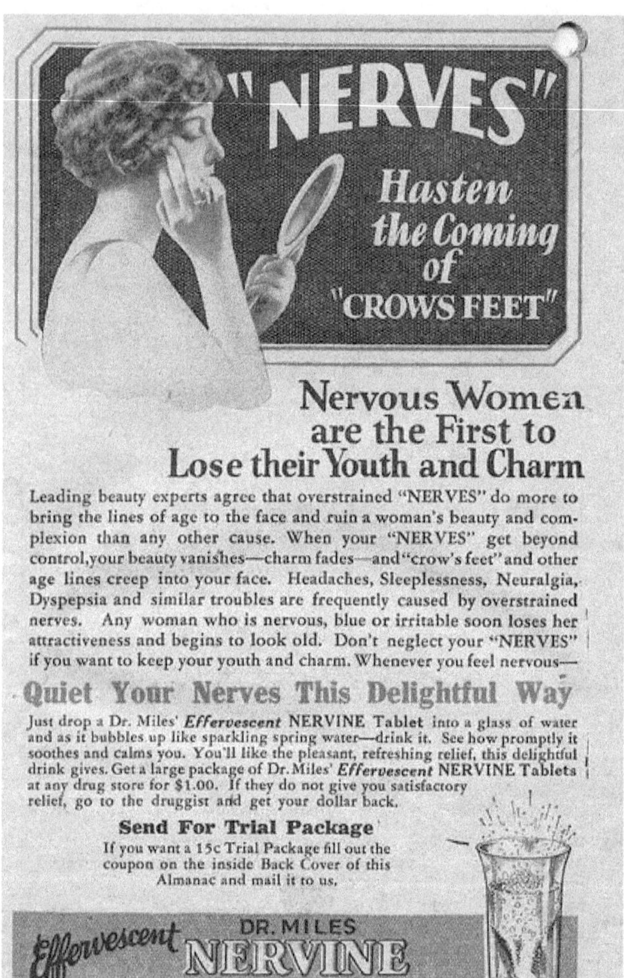

Given some of the previous ads we've seen,
I'd be very nervous about what's in this stuff.

Worse

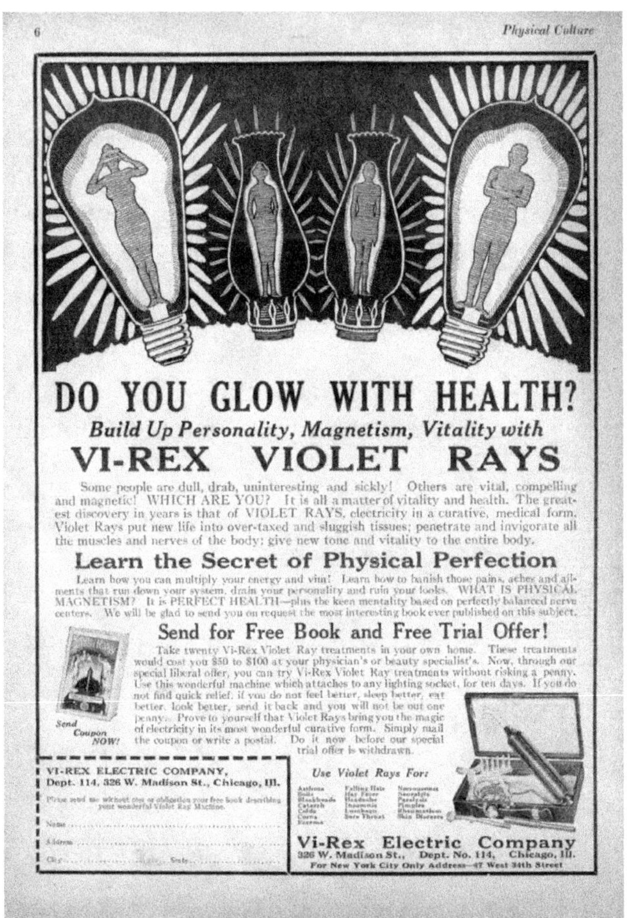

If the shaking chair didn't work,
now you can try electrocuting yourself.

Practical Page:

<u>Word of Mouth</u>
The Bible says to show honor where honor is due (Romans 13:7). Praise those who have helped you, and when possible, do it in front of others. This is especially important regarding long-term help such as from a spouse or close friend. Human nature leans toward mentioning our latest frustration rather than remembering sacrifice made over the long seasons of illness.

If there is something good to praise, say it! Public appreciation can be highly meaningful and motivating to a weary helper.

137

For He satisfies the longing soul,
and fills the hungry soul with goodness.
Psalm 107:9

CONCLUSION

It does not matter how great the pressure is.
What really matters is where the pressure lies —
whether it comes between you and God,
or whether it presses you nearer His heart.
J. Hudson Taylor[xxii]

The first book in the *Sick & Tired* series began late one night when I'd taken a huge dose of prednisone, couldn't sleep, and my mind was running at warp speed. It seems fitting that the final book should end with the same. No announcement of a magic cure. No driving off into the sunset (not until Heaven anyway—more likely driving to another appointment!), no promises that if you try this product or program then snap, your problems will be over.

No, this book, like the others, is by and for those of us who still fight, falter and fail…and keep going. Maybe we're not going quickly, or anyplace more exciting than the pharmacy, but we're going. We've learned to stick it out, endure, bear our burdens and sometimes each others. Most of all we've learned how to depend fully, helplessly, desperately on God in ways healthy, energetic, fulfilled-feeling people never can. In that upside-down way Jesus loves, they're the ones missing out.

Suffering can be a high calling, if we accept it as so. It can also be a mud pit, if we wallow in it. Or the path to destruction if we let it leech us of joy. Amazingly, in one of God's wondrous created laws of the human spirit, though we can rarely control our circumstances, we can always control our response to them.

The sicknesses we live with are not our choice, but how we live with them is.

In Uganda, where I lived for nine months, some of the roads were fraught with potholes. Not little bump potholes, holes big enough to eat a car. There was no driving on auto pilot, no nice, comfy Sunday drive outings. It was work and if there was not a good reason, those trips were to be avoided.

For me, one of the worst roads was on the way to language class. I wasn't going shopping or to a picnic. This was important, and there were no better routes. Each time I drove that road, it was worth the struggle to bounce my way along the ridges and avoid the long-horned steers treading over the dirt roadway, and watch to keep out of those destructive holes. It was worth it because I had a purpose at the end. This wasn't a joyride. It was a mission.

Our lives have to take on that same sense of purpose. Sickness, the weariness of it over time, will eat us alive if we aren't paying attention. There are bumps and ridges and detours and distractions and waiting, waiting, waiting for answers that may never come. If we're to survive this road with any kind of joy, it's going to have to be intentional.

Why are we here? What's the point of our lives? If you don't know, read the book of John in the Bible. If you do, live like it!

I wouldn't make it without the love and perfect understanding that Jesus Christ gives to me, and the eternal hope of a place where there is no crying and no pain (Revelation 21).

It is fitting to end this series on prednisone with my mind running amuck, but even better to end on the surety that nothing in this life is wasted, not one thing, if all belongs to Jesus.

With that hope, that purpose, that reason to rejoice, I say farewell. Sincerely, I do hope you fare well in all things. Sure, I hope you find a diagnosis, treatment, answer, and feel better soon. But that can't be the ultimate hope, because if it was, some of us would need to throw this away and give up.

Fare well in all the ways that truly matter. Your soul. Your mind. The place where you decide what to live for, what kind of example to be, and what legacy you want to leave behind.

Today, and all the days ahead – good and bad – may you fare well.

Keep going.

You can do this.

Hang on.

Don't give up.

Choose hope.

I'm cheering you on.

Do not be afraid. Stand still,
and see the salvation of the Lord....
The Lord will fight for you,
and you shall hold your peace.
Exodus 14:13b, 14

Seasons

My favorite place is the Blue Ridge Mountains of North Carolina, where spring, summer, fall and winter are distinct, and each beautiful in its own way.

Winter tends to be listed at the end of the year. But it's also the beginning of the next year. During the winter season, the landscape can look desolate, abandoned, void of life, hopeless.

You may be in a winter season with your health right now. Please remember that spring always follows winter. Always. And that empty silence is above ground only. Beneath the surface, much is happening. Life is building, being nourished, preparing for the day when the sun comes back out and it can reach upward and begin anew.

Your season may be very hard right now, but it is a season. For all of God's children, no matter how difficult or painful the current season, we can be sure it is temporary. Spring, new life, resurrection, all are coming, whether soon here in this life by God's grace in delivering us, or forever in the next by His love in giving us eternal life with Him.

If it is winter for you right now, hunker down, snuggle up in the palm of His hand, and rest with hope. Spring is coming. What is seen is not all that is.

Now may the God of hope fill you with
all joy and peace in believing.
Romans 15:13a

The mind controls so much of the body.
We are much more than flesh and blood;
we are complex systems.
Patients do better when they have faith
that they're going to do better.
That's why I always tell my patients
and their families not to
neglect their prayers.
There's nobody I don't say that to.

Ben Carson[xxiii]

Bad

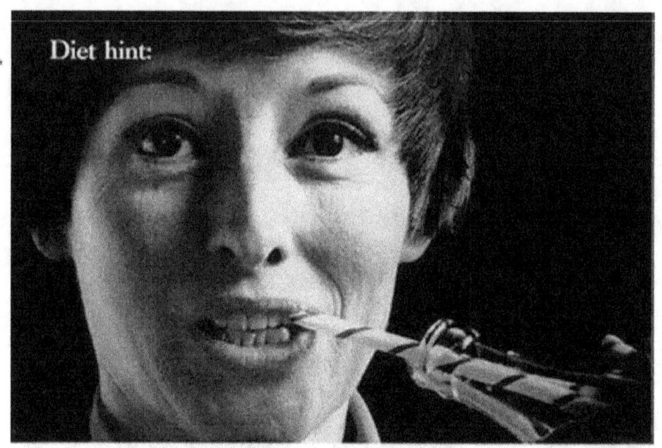

Sugar just might be the
willpower you need
to curb your appetite.

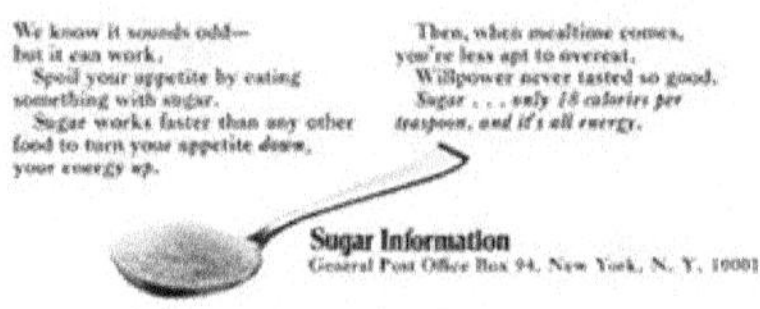

xxiv

This was probably believable to all those people
given 7-Up in their baby bottles.

146

Worse

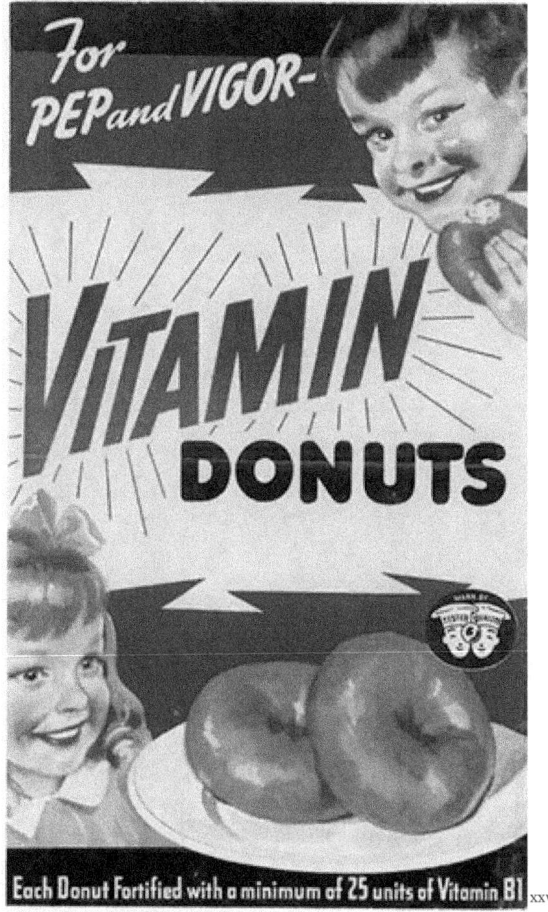

xxv

If only…

Truths to Remember from this Series:

1. You are not alone.
2. People will mess up. So will you.
    Move on.
3. It's not your responsibility to convince
    everyone your illness/symptoms are
    valid.
4. Give yourself and others to God.
5. Let yourself be helped.
6. Less ability does not mean less worth.
7. You are more than your illness.
8. God has a plan for your life.
9. God loves you deeply.
10. Laughter truly is good medicine.
11. Joy is a choice. Choose it!

If I have the stuff inside me
to make cocoons—
maybe the stuff of butterflies
is there too.''
Trina Paulus[xxvi]

I would have lost heart,
unless I had believed
that I would see
the goodness of the Lord
in the land of the living.

Wait on the Lord;
be of good courage,
and He shall strengthen your heart;
wait, I say, on the Lord!
Psalm 27:13-14

APPENDIX A

What Helps Keep Us Going

From Marie:

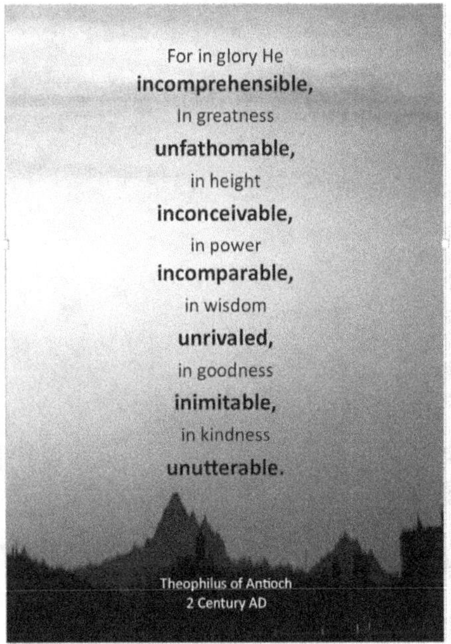

This quote hangs over my desk where I see it every
day. It is my daily prompt to keep an eternal
perspective and to remind myself that
this life is just a blip on the screen of eternity.
God has everything under His sovereign control,
and I can trust that He has a purpose
for my chronic illness.

From Sarah:

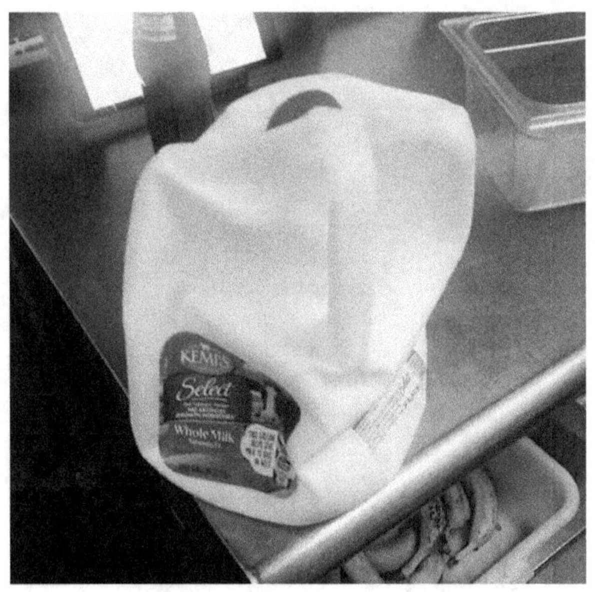

My Ehlers-Danlos Syndrome
depicted by a milk carton!
I saw this and it made me laugh so I took a photo.
I save such pictures to go through on bad days.
Anything that makes us smile helps!

From Me:

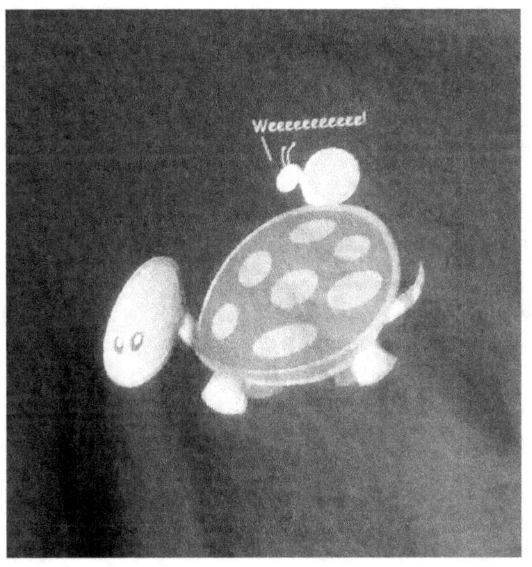

The above is on a shirt I wear to remind me that
it's all about perspective. I have quite a few snails
in my house—not real ones!—to remind me it's okay
to be slower. I'm only expected to be
at the speed I'm designed for and equipped
for in this season of my life.

From Me:

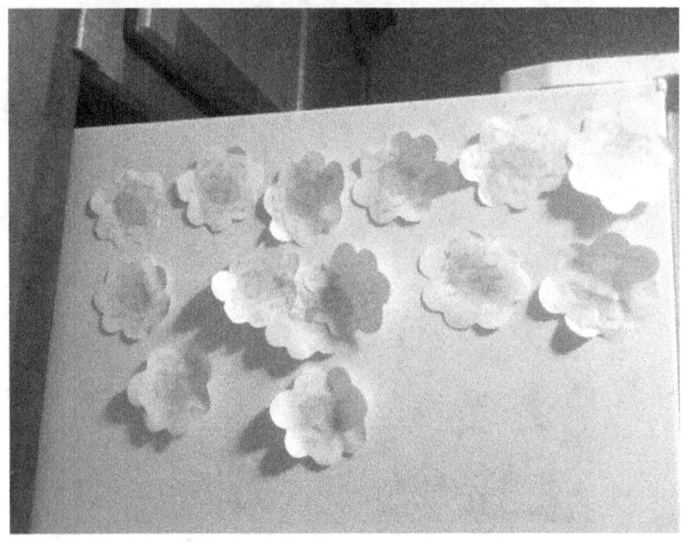

Statements of truth written on flower-shaped
sticky notes that I put on my fridge.

From Sarah:

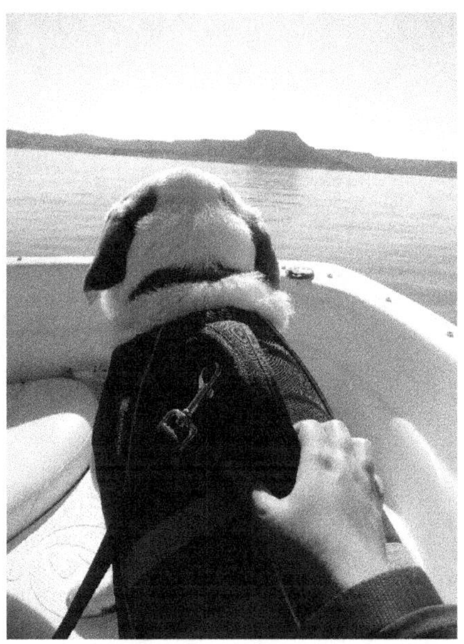

This picture of my pup is motivational for me.
He's terrified of water. Yet here he is, on a boat,
bravely embracing the adventure before him.
Mostly because I'm right there
with him and he trusts me.
Life can be simultaneously scary/intimidating
and fun, and it's OK to embrace both. Why? Because
Jesus is right there with me and I trust Him.

APPENDIX B

Book Recommendations From Us

Anita

The Choice by Dr. Edith Eger

Written by a Holocaust survivor, this book profoundly impacted my outlook on my own situation. While you may have no choice about the events that take place or the things that happen to you, you DO have a choice in how they impact your outlook on the rest of your life. You can wallow in misery, or find something golden. She made me take a hard look at my own attitude, and I have since worked to find positive sparks of joy and hope in each day.

Laura K.

UnShakable Hope by Max Lucado

It gives me encouragement that no matter what storm I am facing, I have a big God who is always there to hold me, even carry me when I can't carry myself. I always have hope in Christ.

Marie:

Hinds Feet on High Places by Hannah Hurnard

This little book changed the way I looked at suffering. Across the years I have read it many times, and have gifted it to many friends who were suffering themselves. The story is an allegory about a crippled young shepherdess named Much Afraid, who lived in the Valley of Humiliation. She longed to follow the Chief Shepherd to the High Places. Oh, what a glorious ending there is to the story! I learned to praise my Shepherd not *in spite of* my MS, but *for* my MS, for I was learning surrender and faith in my Lord.

Anita:
Inner Wisdom by Louise Hay
This short book of daily meditations was recommended to me by a friend. The positive affirmations give me a good start to my day.

Kimberly:
Rose From Briar by Amy Carmichael
Given to me by a dear friend with chronic illness. The book is letters from Amy during her years of being bed-ridden and in pain. I appreciated her acknowledgement that most books for people with sickness are written by the well, and so offered her letters in understanding and transparency. Her spiritual perspective is beautiful.

Sarah:
A Place of Healing: Wrestling with the Mysteries of Suffering, Pain, and God's Sovereignty by Joni Eareckson Tada
This was a very helpful book for me once the reality of chronic illness set in for me. You know, that realization that this isn't going to go away and life won't ever be like it was. This book helped me to

walk through my understanding of suffering in life, and to realize that it isn't necessarily a bad thing to be avoided or a punishment. And it helped me to better understand God's character, His mercy, and that He doesn't enjoy watching us suffer but instead is grieved with us.

ACKNOWLEDGMENTS

How wonderful God is, that He can take my need to write truth and lessons learned for myself, and use it to encourage and help others also.

This final book in the series was the most fun to create, and likely the least organized! It felt a little like leftover stew – piling in all the things that hadn't been said yet in the previous books. One thing that pulled everything together in a special way, however, was the community of people who joined me, sharing their own stories and reminding us all, me included, that we're not alone in our strange sufferings, or in our need for understanding, validation, and hope. Sincere thanks to the team of writers: JD, Laura S. and Laura K., Elaine, Anita, Sarah, Ethel, Tanya, Patricia, K, Phyllis, Marie, and Jacqueline. Your investment, transparency, and insights made this book truly feel like a visit with friends.

Big thanks also to those much-needed beta readers, who find those sneaky typos and give important feedback. Not being a right-brainer, I count on you to make me sound smart!

Future thanks to those who put reviews on Amazon, share on social media, or tell others about this series. You passing on these books or sharing about them with friends is better marketing than anything I could do!

It feels strange finishing this series, as if we are saying goodbye, but I think the friends made along this Sick & Tired journey are going to stay long after the books have gotten old and floppy, and the pages yellowed.

Very best wishes to you, with thanks for the encouragement you have been to me.

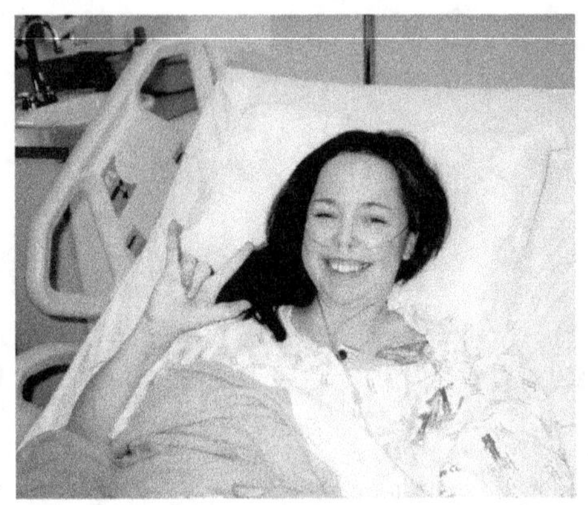

ABOUT THE AUTHOR

Now a brain-surgery survivor, with new conditions including voice box dysfunction and a superhuman sense of smell, Kimberly Rae has over twenty years of experience being sick and tired. Along with her five books on chronic illness, Rae also has written Christian suspense on fighting human trafficking (*Stolen* series and *Shredded* series), and is currently readying to launch the first book in her Small-Town Series, *Coming Home to Hudson*.

Rae lives in Madison, Georgia, with her husband and two children.

Find out more or contact the author at
www.kimberlyrae.com.

Bibliography

[i] coolfunnyquotes.com

[ii] coolfunnyquotes.com

[iii] https://www.healthline.com/health/spoon-theory-chronic-illness-explained-like-never-before#1

[iv] coolfunnyquotes.com

[v] https://www.amazon.com/Some-Days-Youre-Pigeon-Statue/dp/1489702695

[vi] https://www.azquotes.com/author/7479-Barbara_Johnson

[vii] https://www.thethings.com/15-fascinating-and-strange-vintage-ads-for-medical-cures/

[viii] coolfunnyquotes.com

[ix] https://heyjudeparsons.wordpress.com/2014/12/31/captive-of-hope/

[x] https://www.funny-jokes.com/funny/funny_medical_quotes.htm

[xi] https://www.juicyquotes.com/jokes/medical/

[xii] coolfunnyquotes.com

[xiii] coolfunnyquotes.com

[xiv] https://www.leadershipresources.org/the-15-best-james-hudson-taylor-quotes/

[xv] https://www.brainyquote.com/topics/medical

[xvi] https://www.brainyquote.com/quotes/george_carlin_391403

[xvii] coolfunnyquotes.com

[xviii] http://www.thequotablecoach.com/take-my-advice-im-not-using-it/

[xix] https://www.goodreads.com/quotes/50464-stop-worrying-about-the-world-ending-today-it-s-already-tomorrow

[xx] https://www.azquotes.com/author/7479-Barbara_Johnson

[xxi] https://www.funny-jokes.com/funny/funny_medical_quotes.htm

[xxii] https://www.leadershipresources.org/the-15-best-james-hudson-taylor-quotes/

[xxiii] https://www.brainyquote.com/topics/medical

[xxiv] https://www.collectorsweekly.com/articles/the-top-10-most-dangerous-ads/

[xxv] https://www.collectorsweekly.com/articles/the-top-10-most-dangerous-ads/

[xxvi] https://bookquoters.com/book/hope-for-the-flowers